# Dowsing For Joy

*A Manual for Gaining and Maintaining
Your Health and Vitality*

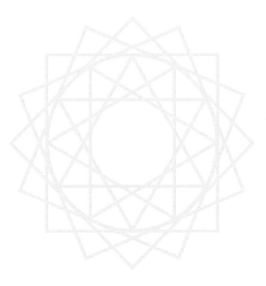

# Joy Lange

Dowsing For Joy
First published in 2012
by Abeon Ltd
81 School Lane, Kenilworth CV8 2GT
www.abeon.co.uk

First Edition : 2012
Design by John Davies
Printed by Warwick Printing Ltd

ISBN : 978-0-9546094-3-6

Please note that Joy Lange does not claim to cure, prevent, diagnose or treat disease. If you have a medical condition please consult the appropriate healthcare professional.

# Contents

# 1. In The Beginning …

Looking back over the years, it is often very difficult to know where our spiritual life begins, and who and what influenced us along this path. As I look back, I really would not have thought that what I am about to say was the start of my journey, leading me on to where I am today.

At the age of thirty, I was married, with four energetic children. My husband, Bern, worked very long hours, so a lot of the time I was dealing with a large house, cooking and cleaning, and taking care of the family, almost single-handed. My days came and went swiftly. I loved growing vegetables, but hardly had time to look after them. Trying to give them some attention, I would often go into the garden, knowing that I would probably only have fifteen minutes to spare before I had another pressing job to do. So I used to set the kitchen timer to buzz at the appropriate time, and I would work like a crazy woman, weeding, planting, digging, just as if my life depended upon it. When my fifteen minutes was up, I rushed onto another job.

It seemed a continual round of running or rushing from one job to another. This became a pattern of how I lived my life. Of course, this eventually took its toll on my health. I became a victim of headaches, and I suffered from migraines that took days to clear. I was always exhausted, and my body constantly ached. I felt tearful a lot of the time, and I found that after a while, I could not face the children in the mornings. It was all too much. To help out, my husband started to cook the children's breakfast, and managed to get them off to school, and the nursery group, so that I could start the day with some kind of peace.

Well, you can tell where this is all leading to. It was not long before I was off to the doctor's surgery, and the prescription for tranquillisers was in my hand, and I began a life of being in a constant daze. I slept a lot, and felt removed from life.

One particular day, when my head was pounding, and I felt particularly bad, I wondered where all this was leading me. This was not a life, it was just an existence, and I did not want to continue this path. I remember crawling under a kitchen chair in the corner of the room. I curled up tight, and sobbed, and begged anything 'out there' to get me from this dark place. It was like going back to the womb. I remember being there for quite a while, and when I had calmed down, I crawled out again, and felt strangely lighter. I made a decision to stop taking the tranquillisers, and felt quite relieved. I wanted more from life than the pills were giving me.

## Martin

It was not long after this event that my in-laws came to visit for a weekend. Martin, my father-in-law was often a pain in the neck. He had a boisterous energy, and often stirred the children up to be as noisy as he was. You would always know where he had been sitting, as there would be numerous scratch-marks on the floor where his restless feet had been. On one occasion he broke the back off one of our chairs as he was demonstrating a wrestling position. So I was not overjoyed by the visit.

During World War Two, Martin was called up into the army, and served in India for four years. He became greatly influenced by their spiritual traditions, and after the war, when he came home, he began to practice yoga. He went on to study more, and joined a yoga class, and went to many healing days and exhibitions, as well as buying numerous books on the subject. None of the family took him very seriously. He was very enthusiastic, and he wanted everyone to live this yogic way of life and to be sensible about eating the right things. So, some of this visit to us that weekend, was about teaching the children to stand on their heads, and to recite the AUM. He then demonstrated the use of a pendulum. It was my first experience of dowsing, and how we all laughed. We were all sure that he moved the crystal himself, and even though he said it was not him moving the pendulum, we were not at all convinced.

Because Martin was so sure that yoga was the answer to many problems, after my in-laws visit, I went along to the library, and borrowed a couple of books on Yoga.  I also noticed that the local authority was putting on a yoga class at a nearby school in the autumn. I made a note of the starting date in my diary. As fate would have it, Richard Hittleman, an American yoga teacher, started a series of yoga sessions on the television in the afternoons, and, coincidentally, it finished just as I needed to leave to pick up the children from school. I joined in with the exercises, and really enjoyed the stretching.

Over the weeks that followed, I noticed that I began to feel better. I did not ache so much, and I certainly felt calmer. My headaches were still there, and the migraine was just as painful, but I coped.

## Classes now

I joined the local authority yoga class in the autumn, and enjoyed the company of other mums, doing the same thing. After about five years of attending the class, three of us mums were asked to stay behind after the class. We all had worried looks on our faces - what had we done ?  We were soon put at our ease, as the principal of the evening class said that she was looking for more yoga teachers to teach other venues, and we had been singled out as possible teachers. They would put us on a training course to gain a certificate enabling us to teach adults, and they would also pay for us to be trained by a national yoga association. It was left that we would give our decisions the following week.

I talked it over with my husband, when I arrived home.  Could I really manage to do this? My mind was in a turmoil.  Did I have the confidence, the energy, or time to do this. My husband said at one point in our conversation "Do you *want* to do this ?" and I suddenly realised that I wanted to do this more than anything. *"Yes I do, but…"*  *"No buts"* he said, *"lets see how we can manage."*

That is how it started. I was now on some kind of a path, and I felt really excited at the prospect of learning new things. I knew that I was more than a wife, and a mother. I reflected on the occasion when I had been at my lowest, maybe  'something' *had* listened to me.

Martin was over the moon at my news, and lent me lots of his books. One of them was on Dowsing. I promised him that I would read it, which I did, several times. I then started to use a pendulum. The book told me to have a 'natural' pendulum, so I made one out of a piece of wood and some newly-spun sheep's wool.  It was not too successful, but I seemed to get some results. I later chose crystal and metal pendulums, and began to get better results.

## New learning

I read much about dowsing for water and energy lines, but I was more drawn to what I could find regarding my family's health. My daughter had suffered from severe eczema from the age of three months, and as she was growing up, the angry red, sore patches all over her body got worse. She was the one that I focused on first. I devised a list of foods and drinks, and gradually worked through these, checking with the pendulum. I was horrified to find that cows' produce was affecting her extremely badly. She was far from happy when we left these out of her diet. Cheese was one of her favourite foods, and of course, finding that chocolate was also a big 'no no', was the final straw. My daughter, because of eczema, and the distress it caused her, was not always a 'happy bunny'. She was often moody, and seemed to get angry at the slightest thing. It was however, very noticeable after a few weeks of the restricted diet, that the eczema was certainly healing, and her moods lessened. We found a source of goats' milk and cheese that she could tolerate, and things improved. I was thrilled. What else could we find ? I discovered that I also was allergic to cows' produce. I have never had eczema, but my migraines disappeared after leaving out the cows' produce. I also noticed that my energy levels improved, which enabled me to cope better with my course work.

I passed my exams, and then went on to teach yoga twice a week in a couple of the local villages. Dowsing was certainly brought into the classes, and I began to teach others to do as I did. It was lovely to see them getting good results too.

I began to get a thirst for learning more. As well as teaching yoga, I trained as a Reflextherapist, and went on healing courses, and trained in counselling. I passed my exams in Hypnotherapy, and attended many crystal workshops. I learnt about Bach Flowers, after which I found Kinesiology, which really fascinated me, because it was just like dowsing.

## Using my new knowledge

Our children grew up, left home, and had their own families. My husband and I moved to a smaller house, and I started working in a therapy centre practicing reflextherapy. I vividly remember my first week of working there. A lady had made an appointment to see me, and was brought in to the centre by her husband. The receptionist told me that the lady (let's call her Mrs A) was having a panic attack in reception, and could I please leave the door open when she came in, and could we have the window wide open. She had a great fear of being closed in. I agreed, even though it was the middle of winter, and it was a freezing cold day.

Mrs A came in, and was visibly shaking. She said that she had heard that reflextherapy could help her to relax, and that was why she had decided to come. She had not been out of the house for many months, and seemed to be afraid of everything. After the treatment, she did look a bit calmer, and I told her of the areas that I had picked up on her feet. One particular area was her stomach. She said that she often felt quite nauseous, and had to make frequent visits to the toilet. I asked whether I could do an allergy test on her as foods and drinks often caused the symptoms that she had, and would she mind if I cut a snip of her hair to work on when I got home. We agreed that I would see her the following week, and I would let her know my findings.

I took the hair sample home in an envelope, and during that evening I ran through my list of foods and drinks. I dowsed over the envelope, and asked *"Is this person allergic to this product."* Cows' produce came up as a very strong allergy, as well as citrus, and a few other things.

The following week, we went through the same process as before, leaving the window and door open. Mrs A was very shaky, and again, was very tearful. Before her treatment, I gave her the list of allergies that I had been working on, and we talked over my findings. She admitted that she did have a lot of the dairy produce, and ate a lot of chocolate. Over the next week she promised that she would leave the items out of her diet, and we would see how she felt.

Mrs A came back the following week, all smiles. She said that today she had actually had the confidence to travel by bus without her husband. She was swinging a Marks & Spencer bag, and said she had not been able to shop for about a year, owing to her fears. She said that after the third day of leaving out the dairy produce, the nauseous feeling had gone and she did not feel so shaky. We no longer had to leave the window and door open in the treatment room.

Coming back to the centre, a month later, Mrs A was a different woman. She smiled a lot, and asked whether I would see other members of her family. The family had seen such a change in her, they were curious as to whether they might also have allergies. She wanted to know how I had isolated the allergies, and would I show her how it was done. I felt a bit anxious as I told her of how I dowsed, but she accepted it without any question, and said it worked, so she felt very happy.

Mrs A went on to get herself a job working for an optician. I would sometimes look through the window where she worked, without her noticing me. She always seemed to be smiling. I felt very pleased with the results of dowsing, and vowed that I would always allergy test my clients before I gave them reflextherapy, so the treatment would be more beneficial.

## Teaching others

More and more people booked into the centre to see me, some of them came just for an allergy test. Amazing really, as I never ever advertised. All my clients came by word of mouth. This confirmed to me that many people were benefitting from my dowsing methods. I was asked many times *"Where did you train to do this ?"*, and when my answer was *"I trained myself"* I was asked to run a course. So, in 1986 I ran my first workshop.

For Part 1 of the course, I concentrated on the Physical level. I re-vamped my list, and added other allergens to my handout, like metals, plastics and environmental products. We dowsed for Bach Flower remedies, sent absent healing, and found that it was possible to heal certain areas of the body via the pendulum. We also dowsed for supplements, herbs and homeopathy.

Part 2, just seemed to follow on naturally. It covered the emotional blocks, and how we could contact feelings from the past, and release them in a symbolic way.

Part 3 was the final stage, and was titled 'Spirituality' where we used colours, signs and symbols to heal.

All these areas just presented themselves to me, without a lot of effort. I used all these areas on myself, which helped me enormously. I felt alive, and full of light. I seemed to have found a wonderful purpose in life and this encouraged my enthusiasm for helping people to heal and to grow. Dowsing, to me, seemed to be the perfect way of achieving this.

## All our journeys

Watching people heal and grow, with these simple techniques, has been amazing. Hearing the differing stories of how a life has been changed is always rewarding. I see the writing of this book as an opportunity to reach out to others to continue the work.

I realise that we all have the answers within us. If I had not moved from that desperate place all those years ago, maybe the story would be so different now. We all have to go through some 'grot', but if we see these difficulties as an opportunity to learn more about ourselves, and yes, asking for help, the rewards are tremendous, and we become the richer for it.

## Acknowledgements

Thank you John for all your help and advice in writing this book. Without you this would not be written.

Thank you to all my very special friends and family that have supported me, particularly over the last couple of years. Your love, care and support has helped me beyond measure. I can now move forward into untroubled waters.

To Bern, who was a fountain of wisdom and knowledge. You helped me on my path. You are sadly missed, but never forgotten.

Last, but far from least, to Martin, my father-in-law. You showed me a path in the beginning. Your influence has made me who I am today.

**Joy Lange**
*June 2012*

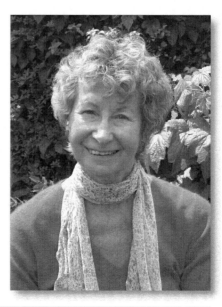

## Tools for Dowsing

With any task that we perform, we need the tools to hand to complete it. In the same way, we need tools to begin our dowsing. For what you will learn over the next few pages, you will obviously need a pendulum, and a pen and notebook will be very useful too. In later exercises you will need coloured felt-tipped pens, sugar pills, and a few small bottles. Of course, one of the most important tools for success is an abundance of patience.

As you begin your journey into dowsing, remember to drink water as you work, as this will help you to get accurate results.

Wishing you a wonderful journey.

# Why Do You Want To Dowse

Stepping into the world of dowsing is an exciting adventure, and helps to open many doors.

I know and admire many dowsers who go out into the countryside and find water, ley lines, earthworks and archaeological remains, and other things associated with the land. I have spoken to people employed in Water and Gas Companies who tell me that dowsers are often employed to find leaks, although it is not generally talked about. Sometimes, these dowsers use metal rods for dowsing, but there are some that use a pendulum.

Dowsing with a pendulum can be used for finding lost objects, clearing negative energy from houses, and clearing geopathic stress, identifying allergies, choosing Bach Flower Remedies, Homeopathic remedies, and Tissue Salts. The pendulum is also used for healing purposes.

Dowsing is not for money gain, and not for reading the future. There must always be a valid need for asking a question. Dowsing should not be used to invade anyone's privacy without permission.

Dowsing is not just for the chosen few, it is an art that anyone can learn to do. The only thing that can stop the pendulum working for you, is that you doubt the results. Like starting anything new, you have to practice a bit to get results. Really believe that you can do this. You would not expect to get on a bicycle and ride it perfectly, the first time. Over many years of teaching hundreds of people to dowse on my courses, I have hardly had one person who could not dowse. So, if you have not dowsed before, this is where you begin your journey.

Most people who attend my courses are very much involved in healing, whether they are Acupuncturists, Chiropractors, Reflexologists, or similar therapies. On one particular course, however, a young man booked in who by trade was a car mechanic and I wondered how he would get on. He rang me a couple of weeks later, and said it was fantastic, as he was able to find faults on cars so much quicker now.

My principal interest is the body and health matters, and helping people to grow and develop. So if this is your goal too, then I am delighted, and will do my best to put help you on this path of health, healing and personal development.

This Workbook is structured into separate sections : Physical, Emotional and Spiritual, and it is important to stress that by dealing with the Physical body first, this prepares us for moving later into the Emotions, and then onto Spirituality. I also want to stress here how important it is not to rush through each of the exercises. Working with each of the sections relating to the Physical could take many weeks, but this is many weeks well spent, enabling the body to become stronger and well balanced. When the time comes for you to move on to the next section, it will feel right for you.

## Choice And Care Of A Pendulum

Choose a pendulum that you are attracted to. Some dowsers like wood, or metal. Others will choose a crystal, or some other gemstone. I have seen dowsers using a ring, or a necklace. All of these work, but you will find the results much better if you have a rapport with your pendulum. The shape can be important too. A conical shaped pendulum works very well, as it seem to move much faster than other shapes. Our aim, when dowsing is to be as quick, and as accurate as possible. We do not want to wait forever for the pendulum to move.

As you use your pendulum more, you will need to keep it clear of negative energy. A simple way of doing this is to wrap the pendulum in red tissue, or red material. Make sure that the purse has a red lining. In the past, I have purchased a red purse, only to find the lining of the purse was white, and found this was not so effective. The energy of red helps to burn off negative energy, so this is ideal for protecting your pendulum. Some people like to wash their crystal in salt water, or allow it to be affected by moonlight. Whatever feels right for you will be good.

# How to Dowse Using A Pendulum

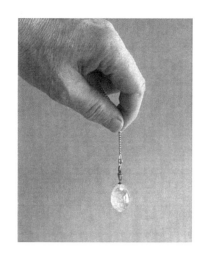

Hold your pendulum between your thumb and first finger, in a fairly relaxed state. To help, you could rest your elbow on the arm of a chair, or a cushion. Empty your mind of thoughts, and start swinging the pendulum backwards and forwards. Do not be too timid about this, as the aim is to have a strong reaction. Now, as the pendulum is swinging, say in your head *"Yes, Yes, Yes"*. The pendulum should change direction. Stop the pendulum swinging, and repeat several times, noting the direction into which the pendulum is swinging.

Now set the pendulum swinging again, and say in your head *"No, No, No"*. Note the direction it is going in now. It should be different from the first movement. Do not be too impatient about this, keep practicing, you will find that when you relax more, there will be a definite difference in the two movements. If you think that it really will not work for you, then that is what will happen. Remaining very positive, believing that the pendulum will give you a *"Yes"* and a *"No"* reaction reaps confident results.

Now you are ready to start. It is important to protect yourself from any negative intervention. Close your eyes. Empty your mind. Now imagine you are filling your head with purple light. Let it overspill into your neck – arms – chest area – lower limbs – right down to your feet.

There may be other ways in which you may like to protect yourself. One of my favourite ways is when I take my shower first thing in the morning. I imagine that the water that is pouring over me is my protection for the day. I find this very quick and efficient.

It is also important to respect your partner's privacy. Everything said in a session must be confidential.

Before you start working with your partner, it is wise to ask these questions :

> *"May I work with this person?"*    (check the response)
> *"Should I do this?"*    (check the response) and
> *"Can I do this?"*    (check the response)

If everything comes up positive *"Yes"*, then you can commence to work with the charts in this Workbook.

It is very important how we ask questions. You could say *"Can I have this?"* and it will come up as being alright, even if it was a poison. What we need to ask is *"Is this good for me?"* So thinking about what you are asking can make quite a difference.

As I was writing this section, I had a telephone call from my daughter. She sounded full of cold, and was sneezing a lot. She was just back from a course, using Hopi Ear Candles, and was worried that the candles were affecting her. She had dowsed over the candles but it seemed as if they were alright, and not affecting her. However, when I dowsed to see whether they were upsetting her, the answer came up as a *"Yes"*. We were confused, as we now had conflicting answers. It then dawned on me that my daughter had dowsed over 'un-burnt' candles. My question was *"Were the candles affecting her?"* This would mean burnt and un-burnt candles. When I asked her to check only for burnt candles, this time the answer then came up as a *"Yes"* so that's what was causing the problem.

So if you are not sure how to ask the question, write it down and look at all angles before you ask.

# Learning To Use Your Pendulum

The following exercises are best performed with a partner. It is often very difficult to dowse for yourself, as we all have pre-conceived ideas about what we want or do not want. For instance, when dowsing for allergies, I, for one, would not like chocolate to come up as an allergy, so having someone dowse for me will be far more truthful than if I dowsed for myself.

If you are a newcomer to dowsing, it really is very important that you are not over-tired. When your energy is depleted it is quite possible to arrive at a wrong answer. This of course, could be very upsetting for someone starting to dowse, when confidence in what you are doing is so important. Being tired could mean that you are dehydrated, so make it a rule to drink water whilst you are dowsing. You will find that it seems to sharpen up the pendulum's response.

Firstly, check out your YES and NO signals. So now, it would be useful to learn to use two other swing signals. Ask the question :

> *"Show me a MAYBE"*

The MAYBE does come up fairly frequently, especially when it is used for testing allergies. A "maybe" is not an allergy, but something that perhaps your partner has eaten or drunk a lot over the last few weeks. Or it could be just a mild allergy. Make a note if this response comes up, and put a question mark beside this item, and go back to it later, so that you can ask a few more questions about it.

Check your YES and NO again, then ask again for your MAYBE. Repeat a few times to be sure of the signal.

Secondly, ask the question :

> *"Show me a DANGER signal"*

This will be a sign that the question you have asked is not for you to know, or it is unwise to proceed. Repeat this a few times until you are sure that this is correct. **Do not try to ignore this answer, but just move on to the next item.** This response does not come up very often, but it is wise to know what it looks like.

## Testing

When working with a partner or client, it is important to remember to respect your partner's privacy by never talking to anyone about what has come up in a session. Your partner is trusting you with, perhaps, very sensitive information. Betraying that trust would spoil that relationship. You will expect the same trust in return when your partner dowses for you.

**Firstly,** protect yourself in your chosen way. Making sure that you will not be disturbed, sit facing your partner, and tune in to him/her. As you proceed, this is done best by looking up from the work occasionally, and looking at your partner and wanting the very best results for them. Try not to **become distracted by** wander**ing** into any conversations while you test. Ask the three questions:

> *"May I work with this person"* (name)    *(check the response)*
> *"Should I do this"*    *(check the response)*
> *"Can I do this"*    *(check the response)*

Once you have received affirmative answers, you can proceed. Start with the *Allergy Test Sheet*. Using, for example, a red pen to mark the allergies, and stating that anything marked in red is to be avoided begin with Cows Produce, and ask the question :

> *"Is this person (or name) allergic to ...*   *Cows Butter*   *(check the response)*
> *Cows Cheese*   *(check the response)*
> *Cows Cream*   *(check the response)*
> *Cows Milk*   *(check the response)*
> *Cows Yogurt*   *(check the response)  etc...*

If the answer to any of these is YES, mark it in red in the box. Continue going down the list in the same way with the other items. If you get a MAYBE coming up on one of the items, clarify the answer by asking the question:

> *"Has this person (name) eaten too much*
> *of this product in the last few days"*   *(check the response)  or*
> *"Should this product be eaten in moderation"*   *(check the response)*

If the product is, for example, wheat, it takes about 3 to 4 days for wheat to pass through the system, and can cause bloating, gassy stomach, even fatigue, as well as other problems, even though it may not necessarily be an allergy. Asking more questions regarding a "maybe" could give you more clues to the sensitivity. For example, ask how many slices of bread could be eaten in one week, without a problem occurring :

> *"Is it one slice per week ..."*   *(check the response)*
> *"... two slices per week ..."*   *(check the response)*

Carry on until you get a YES answer.

   If the product is eggs, how many can be eaten in a week, would it be better to eat an egg when it is cooked in something like a cake, rather than being consumed, like a boiled egg.

   By looking at the *Foods in Balance Sheet*, you may find that your partner is over-acidic. It is a good idea to ask questions about ailments, and to find out what is causing that problem. Having more alkaline foods could be helpful. Over the years of testing for allergies, I have found that the worst offenders are cows produce, and wheat products, but of course, these do not affect everyone. Should a large amount of fruit, onion and tomatoes come up as allergic, it would be wise to check out the Candida Albicans Sheet. Ask the question :

> *"Has (name) got a yeast infection."*   *(check the response)*

If it comes up as a YES, you will need to find out the number of months it will take them to clear the infection. Ask :

> *"Is it one month"*   *(check the response)*
> *"... two months"*   *(check the response)*

Carry on until you get a YES answer. If the pendulum swings for a YES on two months, that is not so bad. A couple of months of the treatment will usually clear it. Up to four, means that your partner has four months work to clear the infection. Your partner will probably have some of the symptoms listed. If it comes up higher, then your partner will have been feeling quite unwell, and possibly suffering from a lot of the symptoms listed.

It is good to check out, perhaps once per month, that it is indeed leaving the system. It usually goes down one place per month, and certainly, your partner will be feeling more energetic as the symptoms leave the body.

NOTE: Once you have completed the Test Sheet, if you can, it is a good idea to make a photocopy so that your partner can take it home with them and review the results.

## Finger Dowsing

Dowsing with a pendulum is all well and good, but there will be times when you wish to dowse, but you do not want to draw attention to yourself. This could be perhaps when you are in the supermarket and you wish to check out a food or drink that may not be suitable for yourself. This is when you can use finger dowsing without others knowing what you are doing.

Make sure that you practice this at home first. Sitting in a relaxed manner, move the thumb and index finger of your dominant hand around and around in a circle. At the same time, say in your head, *"Yes, Yes, Yes"*. Notice what is happening to your thumb and finger.

Now repeat the same process, but this time as you move the index finger and thumb in a circular movement, say in your head *"No, No, No"*. Notice what is happening with your thumb and index finger now.

The responses may be different for some people, but *"Yes"* is often a very smooth movement, and "No" is often a very 'sticky' kind of movement. Get to know what your own signals are by practice. Repeat this exercise several times until you are absolutely sure of the difference between your *"Yes"* and *"No"* responses.

When you are quite happy with your results, use this method of dowsing to check out a few food sensitivities. Hold a piece of food or a drink in one hand, and start the thumb and index finger of the opposite hand moving into a circle, and at the same time saying "Is this good for me?" Also check out a food or drink that you know is not good for you, and notice the response to this.

I use this a lot when out and about, but I have my dowsing finger and thumb in my pocket whilst checking something that I am not sure of, so that no-one knows what I am doing. For example, I use this method when I am choosing a wine. Although I only drink white wine, I find that, even though they may be white, there are several wines that are not good for me, so by just placing one finger on the bottle, and asking *"Is this good for me"*, with the other hand in my pocket I do the finger test, with good results.

I must say that I have seen people using a pendulum in, for example, a health food shop, but I really think that dowsing is not for the eyes of others, so keep it as private as possible.

## Preparing A Hair Sample

I have a number of hair samples in my filing cabinet that have been there for many years. If a client rings me to ask me to check something out, when I use the old hair sample to dowse over, it still gives me the right answers.

- Use a lickable envelope. Cut a small piece of hair, or a nail clipping, and put into the envelope.
- Lick and seal the envelope, and write your full name on the front of the envelope.
- This sample can be kept and used whenever needed. You do not need to use fresh hair or nail each time you test, as the energy surrounding these items will continue to be there.

# How The Mind Can Influence The Pendulum

I have already mentioned that tiredness can affect the pendulum results. The pendulum can also be affected by the mind. Wanting a particular outcome to the dowsing can definitely affect the answer. You can experience how this happens by doing the exercise below :

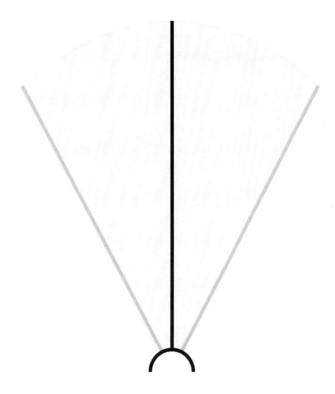

Set your pendulum swinging on the centre line of the diagram, but let your mind concentrate, and look, at the line on the right side. You will notice that the pendulum will swing to that side. Take the pendulum back to the centre line, and then allow the mind and the eyes to concentrate on the line to the left. Once again, you will notice that the pendulum follows the mind.

So, to get accurate answers, it is very important to keep the mind out of the dowsing, to help you focus only on the question you are answering, and the person you are dowsing for.

Look at the person you are dowsing for occasionally, and do not let your mind wander to other things outside the questions you are asking. If you are working with allergies, think of the food you are checking out, and, perhaps, name the person you are working with. So for example, "is Mary allergic to cows milk?" When you ask this question, try to think of a carton of milk.  By doing this, you present a picture of the milk to your partner's energy field, and so as you dowse for the person, you get an accurate answer.

*Teachers open the door*
*but you must enter by yourself*

Chinese Proverb

# I. Physical

A vegetarian diet with a good variety of grains and vegetables, beans and pulses, with fruits that are eaten in the way they are grown, meaning not juiced, puts you squarely on the way to an alkaline diet.

Fats and sugars are the enemies, plus too many wheat-based foods, which break down into sugars, but of course can be eaten in moderation.

I have noticed over the years, working with clients who have allergies, wheat comes up more and more as an allergic food. Wheat is not produced in the way it was in my grandparents' time. The grains of wheat were much rougher then, and worked their way through the system fairly quickly. The grains are processed now, making them softer, which causes them to take time getting through the body. It can take up to 4 days for the wheat to pass through, which means, it rots down on the way, causing a lot of acidity, which in turn will cause bloating, constipation and wind problems, and because this is turned into sugars, we have an abundance of obesity problems too.

Because of processed foods, most of us eat much too quickly. As the foods are soft, we do not chew enough. This in turn stops our foods from not getting digested properly. So we finish up again with more acidity in our system than our body can cope with.

So, chewing thoroughly, eating less of the fatty, sugary foods, and more of the alkaline foods will help us all onto a healthier path.

# Helping You Use Your Dowsing

So you can now dowse, and I am sure you are itching to use the pendulum in a productive way, helping you to become a healthier person.

If you focus in on what you want to achieve from this exercise, it would be helpful to write down what problem you would want to solve. For instance, it could be that you or your partner may be suffering from skin problems, or headaches, or bad moods. Keep this in mind as you work through the Allergy and Diagnostic Test Sheets.

As I have said before, it is so important to realise (especially if you are new to dowsing) not to over-stretch your energies at this time. Doing too much will cause fatigue, which may cause wrong answers. Pace yourself, as this will result in a successful outcome.

Starting with the Allergy Test Sheet, find a partner to work with, or if you are working on yourself it will be far more successful if you work on your hair sample. If you have decided on working with a hair sample, hold this in your hand, and say :

*"Is this person allergic to Cows milk, cows cheese, butter, cream etc ...?"*

By saying 'this person' it really takes the pressure off yourself. Its as if you were dealing with another person, then you won't try to over-rule something that you would like to keep in your diet. Remember, you are working with the Allergy Test Sheet to become a healthier person.

If you are working with another person, get them to specify why they want the Allergy test. Have this in mind as you dowse through the list.

Sit facing your partner. Check your responses, your Yes/No signals. Ask whether you can work with this person.

If all is well, start the work by gradually going down the Allergy Test Sheet and asking :

*"Is (person's name) allergic to Cows milk, Cows Butter Cows Cheese, Cows Yogurt?"*

If any come up, mark at the side with a red pen. Gradually go through the whole sheet, with as little conversation as possible. Try to keep your mind on the list, and on the problem that has caused you to do this Allergy test.

At the end of the list, ask your partner what they thought of the outcome. How much of this product were they consuming? It is important that your partner stops having these foods. Encourage them to leave the offending items out of their diet for a whole week, and then re-assess how they are with the problem they stated they had. It could take a bit longer to experience some change, but having contact with each other will give support to the changes. It is possible that the allergies that were picked up will be permanent, and so alternatives will have to be sought. If alternatives are chosen, it is important to check these too, as these may also affect the person.

# Allergy Test Sheet

Client ........................................    Date ..................................

## Cows

Butter .................. ❏
Cheese .................. ❏
Cream .................. ❏
Milk .................. ❏
Yogurt .................. ❏
Other .................. ❏

## Goats

Cheese .................. ❏
Milk .................. ❏
Yogurt .................. ❏

## Sheep

Cheese .................. ❏
Lanolin .................. ❏
Milk .................. ❏
Wool .................. ❏
Yogurt .................. ❏

## Soya

Beans .................. ❏
Cheese .................. ❏
Milk .................. ❏

## Meats

Bacon .................. ❏
Beef .................. ❏
Chicken .................. ❏
Duck .................. ❏
Game .................. ❏
Ham .................. ❏
Lamb .................. ❏
Liver .................. ❏
Pork .................. ❏
Paté .................. ❏
Quorn .................. ❏
Sausage .................. ❏
Turkey .................. ❏
Venison .................. ❏
Other .................. ❏

## Fish

Cod Liver Oil .......... ❏
Fish in Brine .......... ❏
Fish in Oil .............. ❏
Oily Fish .............. ❏
Shellfish .............. ❏
White Fish .............. ❏

## Grains

Barley .................. ❏
Corn .................. ❏
Maize .................. ❏
Millet .................. ❏
Oats .................. ❏
Rice .................. ❏
Rye .................. ❏
Wheat .................. ❏

## Beverages

Beer .................. ❏
Chocolate .............. ❏
Coffee .................. ❏
Lager .................. ❏
Spirits .................. ❏
Squash .................. ❏
Tea
  Bags .................. ❏
  Fruit .................. ❏
  Loose .............. ❏
Water
  Bottled .............. ❏
  Fizzy .................. ❏
  Tap .................. ❏
Wine
  Red .................. ❏
  White .................. ❏
Other .................. ❏

## Vegetables

Asparagus .............. ❏
Aubergine .............. ❏
Bamboo Sprouts ......... ❏
Beetroot .............. ❏
Broccoli .............. ❏
Brussels Sprouts ...... ❏
Cabbage
  Red .................. ❏
  White .................. ❏
Carrots .............. ❏
Cauliflower .............. ❏
Celery .................. ❏
Chives .................. ❏
Courgette .............. ❏
Cucumber .............. ❏
Garlic .................. ❏
Kale .................. ❏
Leeks .................. ❏
Lettuce .................. ❏
Onions
  Raw .................. ❏
  Cooked .............. ❏
Parsley .................. ❏
Parsnips .............. ❏
Peas .................. ❏
Peppers .............. ❏
Potatoes
  Baked .............. ❏
  Crisps .............. ❏
  Fried .................. ❏
  Jacket .............. ❏
  Plain .................. ❏
Pumpkin .............. ❏
Radish .................. ❏
Runner Beans ............ ❏
Spinach .............. ❏
Tomatoes
  Fresh .................. ❏
  Tinned .............. ❏
Watercress .............. ❏
Other .................. ❏

## Fruit

Apples
- Sharp .................. ❏
- Sweet .................. ❏

Apricot .................... ❏
Avocado ................. ❏
Banana ................... ❏
Blackberry ............. ❏
Blueberry ................. ❏
Cherry ................... ❏
Coconut ................. ❏
Currant .................. ❏
Date ...................... ❏
Dried Fruit ............. ❏
Fig ........................ ❏

Grape
- Green .................. ❏
- Red .................... ❏

Grapefruit ................. ❏
Gooseberry ............. ❏
Kiwi ...................... ❏
Lemon ................... ❏
Lime ...................... ❏
Mango ................... ❏
Melon ................... ❏
Nectarine ................. ❏
Orange ................... ❏
Peach ................... ❏
Pear ...................... ❏
Pineapple ................. ❏
Plum ...................... ❏
Prune .................... ❏
Raspberry ............. ❏
Redcurrant ............. ❏
Rhubarb ................. ❏
Raisin .................... ❏
Satsuma ................. ❏
Starfruit ................. ❏
Strawberry ............. ❏
Sultana .................. ❏
Tangerine ................. ❏
Other .................... ❏

## Other Foods

Beans .................... ❏
Chocolate Bars ........ ❏
Eggs ...................... ❏
Herbs .................... ❏
Marmite ................. ❏
Mushrooms ............. ❏
Nuts ...................... ❏

Oils
- Olive .................... ❏
- Safflower ............. ❏
- Soya .................... ❏
- Sunflower ............. ❏

Pulses ................... ❏
Salt ...................... ❏
Seeds .................... ❏
Spices ................... ❏
Sugar .................... ❏
Tahini ................... ❏

## Environmental

Plastics ................... ❏

Metals
- Aluminium ............. ❏
- Amalgam (teeth) ...... ❏
- Brass ................... ❏
- Chrome ................. ❏
- Copper ................. ❏
- Gold .................... ❏
- Iron .................... ❏
- Lead .................... ❏
- Mercury ................. ❏
- Platinum ................. ❏
- Silver ................... ❏
- Tin ...................... ❏
- Zinc .................... ❏

## House & Garden

Air Freshener .......... ❏
Clothes Conditioner ... ❏
Detergent ................. ❏

Dust
- Garden ................. ❏
- House .................. ❏
- Mites ................... ❏

Grass
- Cut ..................... ❏
- Seed ................... ❏

Household Cleaner ... ❏
Minerals ................. ❏
Perfume ................. ❏
Pollen ................... ❏
Potpourri ................. ❏
Pot Plants ............. ❏
Prescribed Drugs ..... ❏
Shower Gel ............. ❏

Sprays
- Deodorant ........... ❏

Polish ................... ❏
Toilet Block ............ ❏
Toothpaste ............. ❏
Vitamins ................. ❏
Other ................... ❏

## Animals

Cat ...................... ❏
Cow ...................... ❏
Dog ...................... ❏
Gerbil ................... ❏
Hamster ................. ❏
Horse ................... ❏
Rabbit ................... ❏
Sheep ................... ❏
Other ................... ❏

## Feathers

Bird ...................... ❏
Duvet ................... ❏
Pillow ................... ❏

---

## Notes

---

# Working with the Diagnostic Sheet

After identifying the food allergies, you can now move on to the *Diagnostic Sheet* with your partner. Again, check your YES and NO signals. Check the response to the three fundamental questions. If all is well, move on to the chart, and starting with the first item, ask:

"*Is (name) affected by Earth Lines ?*"

If "*Yes*", put a mark at the side, and come back to it later. Continuing, ask:

"*Is (name) affected by Microwave ?*"

Again, if "*Yes*", mark at the side.

Continue going through the lists, marking where appropriate The marked areas will show where some work can be done. We must always remember though, that we will not have the answer to everything. There will be areas that will fall into the hands of the professionals, and clients should be advised to seek their help where appropriate. We are not the answer to everyone's problem.

   After you have checked through the list, and highlighted the problem areas, you can now concentrate on finding some answers.

| | |
|---|---|
| EARTH LINES | See sheet on "Clearing Negative Energy from property" Follow the instructions. |
| MICROWAVE | Get the microwave checked out for leakage. Is it a very old microwave ? Or is my partner too near to the microwave when it is being used? |
| COLOURS | Whilst some colours can upset a person's energy field, others can be helpful. For instance wearing a lot of black is like living in a dark tunnel. Go through the spectrum until you find the colour that is upsetting, or is helpful, for your partner's system. If it is helpful, encourage your partner to wear this colour, or to put on coloured underwear. |
| NOISE | Ask : Is this to do with the radio, television, machinery, traffic, or something else? Can something be done about this? |
| TELEVISION | Ask : Is (name) watching too much television. Is it too scary, or are they watching too late at night, or sitting too close to the set. |
| COMPUTER | Ask : <br> "*Is (name) working too late on computer, or for too long?* |
| MACHINERY | Similar to Noise. Ask if there is something that can be done about this? |
| PSYCHIC | Is there something around that needs to be moved on? [*Physical: 'Clearing Negative Earth Lines / Psychic Energy from Property'*] Or maybe they need to read something on understanding psychic energy. |
| CHEMICAL | Ask : Is this a chemical that may be used for cleansing the body, such shampoo, conditioner, deodorant, or for cleaning |

the home, or being used in the garden. Or somewhere else. [*Physical: 'Ingredients to Avoid in Personal Care Products'* or *'Common Environmental Chemicals'* etc.]

| | |
|---|---|
| RELATIONSHIPS | Is this male, or female? A partner, a friend, or an acquaintance? [*Emotional: 'Cutting The Ties That Bind.'*] |
| KARMIC | This will relate to past lives. [*Emotional* and *Spiritual*] |
| HEREDITARY INFLUENCES | [*Emotional: 'Clearing Miasms.'*] Dowse to find which of these is applicable, and make up Bach Flower remedy to clear. 6 drops of each of the remedies to be taken twice per day for 6 days. Check to see that the Miasm has gone after 6 days. If not, repeat the remedies. |
| HORMONE IMBALANCE | Does your partner need to see a nutritionist, or a doctor regarding menopause, or thyroid, or something else. |
| MENTAL IMBALANCE | [*Emotional: 'Emotional Stress Release'*] |
| BACTERIA | Check where this is. Ask questions of your partner. Would Echinacea help, or Golden Seal, or Vitamin C, or something else. What is it ? |
| ALLERGIES | Is there something that you may have missed, or was not on the Allergy Sheet? |
| BLOCKS TO HEALING | [*Emotional: 'Emotional Stress Release'*] |
| THERAPY | Would your partner be helped with any of the listed therapies? |
| PHYSICAL CAUSES | Ask *"Am I looking for a cause?"* If the answer is "Yes" go down the *Physical Cause* list and see which one(s) may be applicable. |
| OSTEOPATHIC LESIONS | Which of the vertebrae is/are out? Check to see if it relates to any symptoms your partner may be experiencing.<br>*"Does (name) need an Osteopath or a Chiropractor?"*<br>*"Is the problem muscular?"* If "Yes"<br>*"Does (name) need Bowen Technique, or Remedial Massage?"* |
| CONSTITUTIONAL REMEDIES | These are Homeopathic Remedies that are helpful if you are feeling under the weather, and relate to your emotional type. Dowse to see which one is your partner's type. |
| DISEASE | Does your partner need medical help? |
| ACCIDENT AND INJURY | [*Emotional: 'Emotional Stress Release'*] |
| WATER | Many people are dehydrated. Check which area is causing this problem. |
| MERIDIANS | [*Physical: 'Meridians'*] Check to see what could be helpful in the way of diet. Or perhaps a colour. |
| TISSUE SALTS | Dowse to see which one may be needed, and for how long. [*Physical: 'The Twelve New Era Tissue Salts'*] |
| CHAKRAS | [*Physical: The Importance Of The Chakras'; 'Balancing The Chakras Through Dowsing'*] |

# Diagnostic Sheet

Client ........................................ Date ...................................

## Radiation in Home/Work
Earth Lines ............... ❑
Microwave ............... ❑
Colours ..................... ❑
Noise ........................ ❑
Television .................. ❑
Computer .................. ❑
Machinery ............... ❑
Psychic ..................... ❑
Chemical .................. ❑
Relationship ........... ❑

## Karmic Influences
Physical ................. ❑
Emotional .................. ❑
Spiritual ................. ❑

## Hereditary Miasms
Psoric ..................... ❑
Syphilis ..................... ❑
Tuberculosis ........... ❑
Gonorrhea ............... ❑
Cancer ..................... ❑

## Allergies
Foods ..................... ❑
Drinks ..................... ❑
Metal ........................ ❑
Environmental ......... ❑
................................
## Mental Imbalance
Depression ............... ❑
Mania ..................... ❑
Boredom .................. ❑
Anger ..................... ❑
Fear ........................ ❑
Guilt ........................ ❑
Hysteria .................. ❑
Jealousy .................. ❑
Anxiety ..................... ❑
Sadness .................. ❑

## Hormone Imbalance
Physical ................. ❑

## Bacteria
Physical ................. ❑

## Blocks to Healing
Grief ........................ ❑
Accident .................. ❑
Shock ..................... ❑
Surgery ................. ❑
Drugs ..................... ❑
Concussion ............... ❑
Bacteria ................. ❑
Cortisone ................. ❑
Alcohol ..................... ❑
Vaccination ............... ❑
Smoking .................. ❑
Not wanting to get well ❑
Other ................. ❑

## Therapy
Acupuncture ........... ❑
Aromatherapy ............ ❑
Diet reform ............... ❑
Stress Release ......... ❑
Vitamins ................. ❑
Minerals ................. ❑
Bowen ..................... ❑
Reflexology ............... ❑
Chiropractic ............... ❑
Osteopathy ............... ❑
Massage ................. ❑
Colours ................. ❑
Reiki ........................ ❑
Hypnotherapy ............ ❑
Crystals ................. ❑
Metamorphic ............ ❑
Healing ................. ❑
Affirmations ............... ❑

## Physical Causes
Subluxation ............... ❑
Rotation right / left ...... ❑
Arthritic ..................... ❑
Impinged nerve ......... ❑
Muscle congestion ...... ❑
Lymph imbalance ...... ❑
Ileocaecal valve ......... ❑
Tuberculosis ........... ❑
Houston Valve ............ ❑
Connective tissue ...... ❑
Soft / bony tissue overgrowth ❑
Tumour ..................... ❑
Candida ................. ❑
Myalgic Encephalomyelitis ❑

## Osteopathic Lesions
C0 ......................... ❑
C1 ......................... ❑
C2 ......................... ❑
C3 ......................... ❑
C4 ......................... ❑
C5 ......................... ❑
C6 ......................... ❑
C7 ......................... ❑
T1 ......................... ❑
T2 ......................... ❑
T3 ......................... ❑
T4 ......................... ❑
T5 ......................... ❑
T6 ......................... ❑
T7 ......................... ❑
T8 ......................... ❑
T9 ......................... ❑
T10 ......................... ❑
T11 ......................... ❑
T12 ......................... ❑
L1 ......................... ❑
L2 ......................... ❑
L3 ......................... ❑
L4 ......................... ❑
L5 ......................... ❑
Sacrum ..................... ❑
Coccyx ..................... ❑

## Constitutional Remedies

Arg.Nit .................... ❏
Arsen Alb ................. ❏
Aurum Met ............. ❏
Bryonia .................... ❏
Calc.Carb ................. ❏
China .................... ❏
Kali Mur ............... ❏
Calc Phos ............. ❏
Lachesis ................ ❏
Lycopodium ............. ❏
Merc Met ................. ❏
Nat Mur ............... ❏
Nat Phos ................. ❏
Nux Vom ................. ❏
Phosphor ................. ❏
Pulsatilla ................. ❏
Rhus Tox ................. ❏
Sepia .................... ❏
Sulphur .................... ❏
Zincum .................... ❏

## Meridians

Acupuncture Meridian ❏
Governor ................. ❏
Conception .............. ❏
Heart ....................... ❏
Small Intestine ........ ❏
Circulation Sex ........ ❏
Triple Heater ........... ❏
Spleen .................... ❏
Stomach ................. ❏
Lung ....................... ❏
Colon .................... ❏
Kidney .................... ❏
Bladder .................... ❏
Liver ....................... ❏
Gall Bladder ........... ❏

## Disease

Neurological ............ ❏
Diabetes ................. ❏
Malignancy ............. ❏
Virus ....................... ❏

## Accident and Injury

Physical ................. ❏
Emotional ................. ❏
Spiritual ............... ❏

## Water

Dehydration .............. ❏
Excess Tea/Coffee/Coke/Chocolate ❏
Bedding, atmosphere - too warm ❏

## Tissue Salts

No. 1 Calc. Fluor ...... ❏
No. 2 Calc. Phos. ...... ❏
No. 3 Calc. Sulph ...... ❏
No. 4 Ferr. Phos ...... ❏
No. 5 Kali. Mur ........ ❏
No. 6 Kali. Phos ...... ❏
No. 7 Kali. Sulph ...... ❏
No. 8 Mag. Phos ...... ❏
No. 9 Nat. Mur ........ ❏
No.10 Nat. Phos ...... ❏
No.11 Nat. Sulph ...... ❏
No.12 Silica ............. ❏

## Chakras

Crown .................... ❏
Third Eye ................. ❏
Throat .................... ❏
Heart ....................... ❏
Solar Plexus ........... ❏
Sacral .................... ❏
Base ....................... ❏

## Notes

# Vitality Today

Check with the person you are working with how they are feeling at the start of the session, by dowsing over the chart below, and then compare it with how they feel at the end.

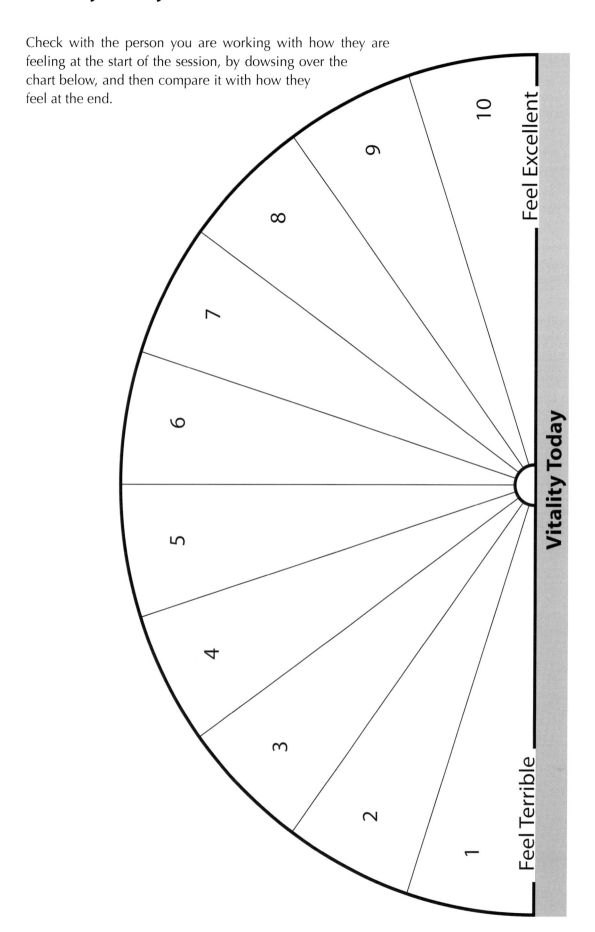

# Healing The Body With Dowsing

Whilst on a Reflextherapy Training Course in 1986, I became rather cross with some of the people who were taking part. We were all practising by treating each other with the therapy that we were learning. For years before this event, I had had a cyst under one foot, and whilst this had never bothered me, it was soon noticed by whoever was treating me. All kinds of comments were made as to what it was all about, like congested bowel, or fatty liver and even "was it a cancer?"

As you can imagine, I was really fed-up with all of this, so shortly after, whilst I was away on holiday, I dowsed to see whether I could get rid of this lump. The pendulum swung to *"Yes"*, so I began to ask questions on what I needed to do. After many questions, and checking the answers, it came up that I needed to swing the pendulum in a circle over that area on my foot for two minutes in the morning, and two minutes in the evening, and this would sort the matter out.

As this was a two week holiday, I promised myself that I would do this every day, until I went home. After about the third day, the area on my foot became rather red and sore, which it had never done before. I was a bit anxious, but continued with the exercise. Over the following days it became even more red, and then suddenly it just disappeared altogether, never to return. It seemed that it had just burnt itself out.

If I have ever had any other minor ache or pain since this time, I treat the problem in the same way and it still works for me.

If you are attempting to use this exercise, ask for your 'healing mode.' My pendulum goes into a circle for this, but it could be something completely different for you. My good friend, Jo, has an unusual healing mode. Her pendulum is very still for a moment when over a sore area, and then vibrates at a tremendous rate when healing. This has produced a lot of success for her, both physically and emotionally. As soon as her pendulum changes direction and starts swinging, she stops the healing.

Always remember the questions you need to ask before you do this exercise, even if it is for yourself :

| | |
|---|---|
| *"May I work with this person" (name)* | *(check the response)* |
| *"Should I do this"* | *(check the response)* |
| *"Can I do this"* | *(check the response)* |

# Oriental Face Diagnosis

This chart is not one to dowse over, it is for observation. I have found it to be very useful in helping to diagnose what is going on with the person I am working with. It is possible to tell where there are blockages, and where help may be needed.

Yellowing around the eyes could be a toxic liver. A line or a fold vertically between the eyebrows could mean suppressed anger. Flushed cheeks indicate lung stress. Bluish tinge to the end of the nose could be a heart problem. It could show that the person is abusing alcohol, or perhaps having too many sweet foods or drinks. If you are one of those people who enjoy sweets and chocolate, you may find that little spots appear around the Duodenum area shown on the chart. Digestive problems show up as swollen lips.

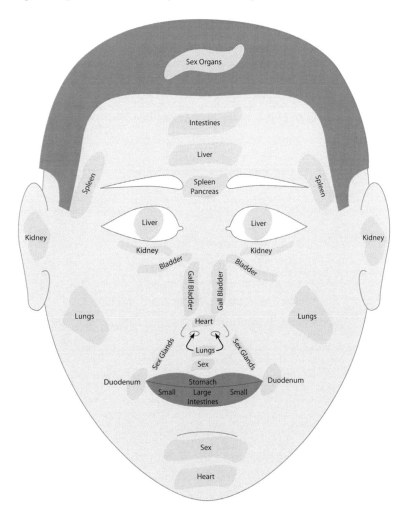

I watched a film showing the life of Elvis Presley, and noted his very swollen lips, and thought at the time he possibly had digestive problems. At the end of the film, it was stated that he had indeed had digestive problems.

So, too many fats and sugars could result in a spotty forehead, and darkening under the eyes, which is the kidney area, could mean that there is a need for more water in the system. Any disorder of the ears could represent excretory functions, regarding the kidney and bowels. This again could be helped by drinking more water.

These areas are just guides to what may be going on, and they should not be taken as absolute truths. If you wish to go deeper into the study of Oriental Face Diagnosis, *"How to See Your Health: Book of Oriental Diagnosis"* by Michio Kushi is the book for you.

# Cleansing The Body

None of us would want to consider the fact that we are often housing unwanted visitors in and on our body. So internal cleansing of the body from time to time is a way of keeping healthy and free of parasites.

Parasites can often affect the intestines, and live within the body for years. They can cause all kinds of health problems. A lot of us visit other countries these days where cleanliness is not a priority. We could also have problems if we handle animals, do not wash our fruits and vegetables thoroughly, and eat raw meats and fish. These all encourage parasites into the body. Some of the symptoms could include anal itching, leaky gut, bloating, cravings for sweet foods, wind, joint pains, burping, teeth grinding, fatigue. Of course, these symptoms may not only be caused by parasites. There could be other health problems, but dowsing to ask the question "Do I/he/she have parasites?" should answer the question.

## To Avoid Parasite Infestation

Wash your hands thoroughly before handling foods. Do not allow pets on kitchen surfaces or in bedrooms. Even if your fruits and vegetables look clean, it is important to wash them thoroughly before eating, not only because they may have parasites, but also because they have been sprayed with chemicals.

## Dietary Recommendations for Parasites

Higher Nature, Burwash Common, East Sussex TN19 7LX offers several products for parasite infections :

| | |
|---|---|
| Paraclens | A combination of artemisia, grapefruit seed extract, barberry, liquorice, ginger, alongside other herbs, specifically designed to eradicate parasites from the body. |
| Citricidal | A grapefruit seed extract that has anti-viral, anti-bacteria, anti-parasitic and anti-fungal properties. Supplementing with this product offers an effective way of eliminating pathogenic organisms from the intestine and the body. |
| Cats Claw Concentrate | A tree bark from the Peruvian rainforest that has anti-parasitic properties. |
| SuperGar | A high potency garlic supplement. Garlic has been a traditional food remedy for intestinal health due to its anti-viral, anti-parasitic, anti-bacterial and anti-fungal action. |
| MSM | Prevents intestinal parasites hooking on to the intestine wall. |

## A Special Note

Intestinal parasites are very perceptive and the eggs will not hatch out into an environment that will kill them. To hatch and kill the eggs and parasites use the Five Step Anti-parasite programme below. The days that you do not take the anti-parasitic formula (Paraclens, Citricidal, Cats Claw or SuperGar) act as hatching days for eggs. Build up to the top dose of your chosen anti-parasitic formula slowly. This will help prevent you experiencing headaches, fuzzy head, nausea etc. from the toxins released as parasites are cleared out.

## The Five Step Anti-Parasite Regime

1. Take maximum dose, every day for 2 months or until symptoms improve, then
2. Take maximum dose, every other day for 2 weeks, then
3. Take maximum dose, every third day for 1 month, then
4. Take maximum dose, once a week for 3 months, then
5. Take maximum dose, once a month for 6 months.

Healing is helped with :

**Aloe Vera** helps to promote a healthy intestine;

**Chlorella** is an algae, rich in amino acids;

**Milk Thistle** to soothe the system.

When you have completed this regime, you might also consider Colonic Hydrotherapy, which helps to cleanse the bowel, and is very good if you suffer from constipation. Any cleansing should be followed by putting natural flora back into the system. Taking a high potency Acidophilus for a month or so would also be helpful.

Chewing foods thoroughly, in a relaxed atmosphere is of utmost importance. Food eaten at the dining table, with other members of the family, with the television turned off, is very good for the digestion, and certainly very good for family relationships.

Try to avoid eating processed foods, particularly wheat products. Too many slices of bread, cakes, biscuits and puddings all slow the system down. The wheat products that are produced today do not contain enough roughage. So when we eat these products, they take longer to get through the body, and could cause constipation.

# Wheat Allergy

Wheat and dairy products quite often come up when dowsing for allergies. This seemed very strange to me at first, until I started looking at them in a different way. In the past, I have thought of these foods as being healthy, but the problem occurs when the natural product is tampered with. Originally, wheat, and the bread that was made from it, was very rustic, in that the grains were very coarse. Eating this bread involved much chewing, and as it was digested, the body extracted the nutrients as it made its way through the many feet of intestines, and usually passed out of the body after a day or so.

In recent times, manufacturers have processed wheat and similar grains in such a way that even wholemeal bread only vaguely resembles the original product. Because of this processing, we do not chew it for so long, and this 'mushy' product goes through the intestines much more slowly as there is very little roughage to help it to do this, and it can take many days to get through the body. It therefore goes through a 'rotting' process, causing a bloated stomach, gas, constipation, and also a build-up of unfavourable bacterial growths. Because wheat breaks down into sugars, we often find that Candida grows in the system, particularly if a lot of sugar is included in the daily diet.

What we have to remember is that by chewing we release chemicals that help us to digest the foods. Watching television as we eat, or eating in a hurry, makes it difficult to digest our foods, and so we then begin to suffer from many symptoms like gas.

One of the other problems our body has to deal with is that preservatives are often added to a lot of the products. The manufacturer wants the foods to have shelf life, so by adding preservatives, the foods appear to be fresh, and seem to last longer. Once upon a time, bread would be stale the day after it was bought. This does not happen now because of the preservatives it contains.

Several years ago I had a funeral director come to me for a consultation. We talked about preservatives. He said that if a body was exhumed after being dead for a few years, there was very little sign of decay, and this was because of all of the preservatives we ingest in our life. I find this a bit scary really.

We may all be affected by wheat products from time to time, which of course may not be a food allergy, but because we have probably consumed too much bread, cakes, biscuits, puddings and pies. There are some people who suffer from inflammatory bowel disease, like Crohn's Disease, sometimes due to low-fibre diets, fast foods and a high consumption of refined carbohydrates and sugars. These people may over-react to wheat products.

People who are Coeliacs will be sensitive to the gluten contained in grains, like wheat, rye, barley and sometimes oats. This could be hereditary. In the past, it was very difficult for these people to get satisfying foods. Manufacturers are now more aware of this fact, and so there are many products on the market for those who need a gluten-free diet.

There are many cases of people suffering from bowel problems. Irritable Bowel Syndrome (IBS) is a phrase that is passed around quite a lot, and I hear it often in my work. The bowel needs to release the debris from what we have eaten. If we do not chew our foods properly, partly undigested foods get locked within the system. If we do not add whole foods into the body, like fibre, bran, nuts and seeds and the like, we are inviting digestive problems. Soft, mushy foods stay within the body, and encourage unwanted bacterial growth.

# Cows Milk Allergy

We are often brainwashed into thinking that only cow's milk can provide our vital need for calcium, but many people are allergic to cow's produce. One of the main reasons for this is that we are taking the metabolism of a larger animal into our smaller body. Goats and sheep are more in keeping with our size.

Average calcium values of dairy and other milks :

| | |
|---|---|
| Cow's milk (Whole) | 120 mg per 100 ml |
| Cow's milk (Skimmed) | 120-125per 100 ml |
| Cow's milk (Semi skimmed) | 120-125per 100 ml |
| Evaporated milk | 290 mg per 100 ml |
| Goat's milk | 120 mg per 100 ml |
| Sheep's milk | 170 mg per 100 ml |
| Soya milk (with added calcium) | 140 mg per 100 ml |

Calcium is essential for building strong teeth and bones, normal blood clotting, nerve functions and enzyme activity. Recent research suggests that having adequate amounts of calcium in early life, and building up a strong skeletal structure may help to prevent osteoporosis in later life. Weight-bearing exercises also help to strengthen bones.

Vitamin D, which is produced by the action of sunlight on the skin, helps with the absorption of calcium by the body, whereas both smoking and excessive drinking of alcohol deplete calcium reserves. There are many other good sources of calcium. These include :

- white or brown bread (fortified).
- Dark green leafy vegetables such as savoy cabbage, spring greens, curly kale, broccoli and spinach.
- Canned sardines or pilchards in oil or tomato sauce are good, providing the bones are eaten.
- Canned baked beans in tomato sauce, red kidney beans, chick peas and lentils.
- Soya beans and tofu, nuts, especially almonds, brazils and hazelnuts.
- Seeds, such as sesame seed and sunflower seeds.
- Dried apricots, dried figs and currants.
- Oats, as in oatbran, porridge and muesli.

In some countries, milk is never used. In places like China, milk is not part of the diet, yet osteoporosis is not one of the diseases that the Chinese people generally suffer from. They do, however, eat a lot of fish and soya products.

There is a school of thought that believes that cow's produce actually blocks the absorption of calcium, and that it can actually cause osteoporosis.

There are many symptoms that can be experienced by someone who is intolerant to cow's produce - Irritable bowel syndrome, headaches, eczema, bad moods, menstrual problems (heavy bleeding) tiredness, lack of energy, asthma, allergic rhinitis (runny nose) sinus problems, stuffy head, loss of smell, just to name a few.

If you suffer from any of these symptoms, a period of one month without cow's produce should see an improvement in your health. Remember that cheese, butter, cream, and yogurt made from cow's milk will also need to be avoided, even though it may be made from skimmed cow's milk.

# Disguised Allergies

Sometimes allergies are difficult to detect. Looking at ingredients on packets is time consuming, but necessary if you have strong reactions to things.

Mrs P has a birthmark on one side of her face, which she disguises with a special make-up. Just before her marriage, she experienced swelling to the other side of her face, which affected her eye considerably. This was worrying, as she obviously wanted to look her best for her wedding. She sought out medical help, and was given several creams and antibiotics, which helped, and the swelling went down. This did not last though, as over a period of time, the swelling came back again, and stayed with her for a week or two, and then disappeared as quickly as it arrived.

On consulting me, I went through the list of allergies, and we found that Mrs P was very allergic to oily fish, and to some shellfish. We found that on each occasion that the swelling had occurred, she had eaten fish, and strangely, this was one of her favourite foods. Thinking that the matter was resolved, I was surprised to have a phone call from her saying that she had not eaten any of the fish I had said was affecting her, but after a meal in a restaurant, the swelling had returned.

As she was on the end of the telephone, I concentrated on her and her voice, and dowsed to find out what had affected her. She went through all the foods she had eaten, one by one, with me dowsing each item. I had a very positive swing when she mentioned the sauce, and we found out later that the sauce had contained anchovies, which are in Worcester Sauce.

Mrs P now makes sure that if she goes out for a meal, or is invited out to friends, she asks what is in the sauce, and with this, she no longer has experienced any swelling of her face.

# Water

I cannot emphasise enough, how important water is. Over many years of seeing clients, I have found that a large number of them have had problems related to dehydration. Some clients have thought that they were drinking enough fluids, but it was not in the form of water. Numerous cups of tea, coffee, or soft drinks may have been consumed in the day, but because these are diuretic, they cause an increase in urine, which obviously results in more fluids being flushed out than are taken in. It is fine to drink tea or coffee, as long as it is not *instead* of water. I would recommend that that no more than four cups of tea or coffee per day are drunk.

When we are dehydrated, we put our mind and body under extreme stress. We cease to function in the way that we should. Toxins build up in the system, which can make us feel tired and irritable. Our concentration is depleted, and we can become confused and then make mistakes. Just think how dangerous this is if, for example, we have a job that requires us to drive long distances, or if we are working in an office where we are making a lot of decisions. Offices will often have air conditioning and central heating, which compound the dehydration problem.

At home, we could have an over-warm atmosphere, and at night we may snuggle under a high tog duvet. The idea of using duvets came from visiting foreign countries where buildings had stone floors and no central heating.  Duvets really have no place in our centrally heated homes with carpet on the floor. The fatigue, or headaches that may be experienced on waking in the morning, could easily be from dehydration. If we overheat our body at night, then get up, pausing only to swallow a cup of coffee before work, we are not giving ourselves a good start to the day.

Water is important for keeping the body's organs functioning properly.  Every tiny cell in the body excretes waste matter, and the cells need water to flush out this waste. Think what it would be like if the dustman did not come around for several weeks to empty the bins. There would be smell, and pollution. Similarly, for our bodies, the consequences are likely to be constipation, spotty and dry skin, apathy, aches and pains in the body, breathing problems and obesity.

Dehydration slows down our metabolism by as much as 3%, so this will not help with losing weight. When we are dehydrated, we often mistake thirst for hunger, and so we may reach for a snack, instead of drinking water. If you are a person who is trying to lose weight, just one glass of water in the evening will help to prevent those midnight hunger pangs.

Water should be sipped slowly throughout the day, enabling the body to effectively utilise the fluid. If water is gulped down very quickly, we find that before long we will be wanting to go to the toilet. It is a bit like watering a plant that has completely dried out. As soon as the plant is watered, it runs through the earth very quickly, and leaves the soil less than moist. If the plant is gradually watered however, the soil can then absorb the fluid and the plant becomes nourished. The same happens when sipping water, gradually the body takes up the fluid, and we become nourished.

So to avoid dehydration, we should drink 2 litres of water per day, sipped slowly. Do not wait until you feel thirsty. By the time you feel thirsty your body is *already* dehydrated.

If you are travelling in the car, make sure that your water is in a glass bottle or a thermos flask. In hot conditions, the chemicals from plastic bottles will poison the water. I have known a few clients who have become very ill with drinking water that has been in their car for a little while.

# E Numbers

Over the years, many children have been brought to me by exhausted parents. The parents often complain that the child sleeps badly, is hyperactive, and can be angry and disruptive. Although sugar can be a cause, in a lot of these cases I have found that the main culprit is an E Number.

It never ceases to amaze me that so many products, that are geared to a child's taste, contain E Numbers. Often, the child appears to be addicted to the food or drink that contains the additive, so it can be very hard for mum to change to another product.

I have had children in my study, climbing up the curtains, scribbling on the wall, and generally being a nightmare. Usually, the mums are very embarrassed, and try hard to control their little demon.

One such occasion I remember very clearly. Mum was actually in tears, and said she really could not cope with things as they were. Her 'little monster' was upsetting the neighbours, hurting his younger brother, and there were complaints from school.

I dowsed over the E Numbers and found several that were seriously affecting the child. Mum admitted that she was using some products that contained these numbers, and that her child was consuming these on a daily basis. She agreed to go through her cupboards and remove all the offending items, and to check the labels of any new items that she bought.

I saw the child again two weeks later, and I could hardly believe that it was the same child. Not only was he nicely behaved, but he sat and read a book right through the session. It had taken Mum a few days to change the offending food and drinks, but by checking the labels, she had found alternatives. Mum was in tears again, but this time, tears of joy.

Like many others, I am an avid label watcher. I like to know what is in the product that I am buying. Although, not all E Numbers are harmful, my experience has shown that we could all be consuming additives without knowing of any potentially harmful side-effects they may have on us. Sometimes, what appears to be an innocent product, could contain a colour or an additive that disrupts our system.

Once, after buying some blackstrap molasses capsules to boost my iron levels, I was surprised to find that it contained E Numbers. I returned it to the health food shop and complained about its contents. I was told that the gelatine capsule was transparent, and because of that, the molasses showed through. By using a dye in the capsule, I was told, it would be more acceptable to the public. *"Not this lady"* I said, and claimed my money back.

So it is wise to check all labels, even on items that you would not expect to include additives. Even health food shops can have some nasties.

The list below contains E Numbers that, in my work, I have found quite often cause a problem for people who are sensitive to colours or additives. See the book *'E for Additives'* by Maurice Hanssen with Jill Marsden, for a comprehensive list.

It is also important to know that it is not only children who have a problem with these. Adults, who seem to run around chasing their tail, or find it difficult to sleep, or who feel angry a lot of the time, may be having a reaction to E Numbers as well.

| E No. | Purpose | Contained in ... |
|---|---|---|
| E102 | Yellow Colour | Drinks, convenience foods, jams, sweets, puddings, smoked fish |
| E104 | Yellow Colour | Desserts, sweets. drinks |
| E110 | Yellow Colour | Preserves, packet soups, sweets, ice mixes, cakes, hot chocolate, jelly |
| E122 | Red Colour | Jelly, sauces, cakes, ice creams, jams, sweets |
| E123 | Red Colour | Gravy granules, tinned pie filling, jelly, soups, tinned fruit |
| E124 | Red Colour | Packet cake mix, dessert topping, tinned fruit, seafood sauces |
| E127 | Red Colour | Tinned fruit, glace cherries, biscuits, chocolate, cooked pork meats, shellfish |
| E128 | Red Colour | Cooked meats, sausage |
| E132 | Blue Colour | Desserts, sweets, biscuits |
| E133 | Blue Colour | Tinned processed peas |
| E142 | Green Colour | Packet and tinned foods, gravy granules |
| E151 | Black Colour | Sauces and deserts |
| E154 | Brown Colour | Smoked fish, crisps, cooked meat |
| E155 | Brown Colour | Chocolate flavours |
| E210 | Preservative | Jams, pickles, fruit juice, dressings, margarine, soft drinks |
| E211 | Preservative | Shellfish, margarine, dressings, drinks, pickles, sauces |
| E223 | Preservative | Alcohol, frozen shellfish, milk products, fruit juices |
| E320 | Preservative | Crisps, biscuits, soft drinks, margarine, cooking fats and oils |
| E321 | Preservative | Margarine, fats, oils, crisps, gravy granules, breakfast cereals |
| E621 | Flavouring | Packet snacks, pork products, stock cubes. |

# Candida Albicans

If many acidic foods come up in the Allergy Test, suspect Candida. The poisons from Candida are extremely acidic. So fruits, onions and tomatoes, for example, will show up as allergic. Often, all or quite a lot of the fruits will show as allergic. This does not mean that the fruits, onions and tomatoes are banned forever. Once the Candida is out of the system these can be put back.

## Potential Symptoms

| | | |
|---|---|---|
| Athletes Foot | Endometriosis | Painful intercourse |
| Abdominal Pain | Excessive menstrual bleeding | Poor memory |
| Acne | Fatigue | Rashes |
| Allergies | Feelings of unreality | Sore throat |
| Bad breath | Frequent urination | Sore gums |
| Bloating | Furred tongue | Spots in eyes |
| Blurred vision | Heartburn | Spots on cheeks and mouth |
| Can't concentrate | Infertility | Swelling/discomfort joints |
| Constipation | Irritability | Tingling and weak muscles |
| Cramps | Loss of libido | Thrush |
| Cystitis | Loss of balance | Tight chest |
| Depression | Migraine | Tingling gums |
| Diarrhoea | Nasal congestion | Vaginitis |
| Dry mouth | Numbness | White spots on tongue |

## Lowered immunity caused by

| | | |
|---|---|---|
| Antibiotics | Damp atmosphere | Stress |
| Caffeine | House plants | Sweet Tooth |
| Cigarettes | Pollution | The Pill |
| Diabetes | Steroids | |

## Candida Assessment and Treatment

Firstly, ask :

> *Has (person's name) got Candida?*

Then ask :

> *How bad is this? On a scale from 1 - 10 where '1' is low and '10' is high, is it '1', '2', '3' etc.*

Based on the answer, the action to take is :

| | |
|---|---|
| From 1-3 | needs about 3 months of leaving out the banned foods and drinks. Take the Acidophilus etc. for this period. |
| From 4-7 | means a longer time. On the Acidophilus etc. and, of course, leaving out the banned foods. |
| From 8 - 10 | monthly checks needed to see that it is reducing. |

**Avoid**

| | | |
|---|---|---|
| All fruits and fruit juices | Coffee | Refined cereals (sugars) |
| Alcohol | Dried fruits | Soy sauce |
| Biscuits/cakes | Fizzy Drinks | Sugary foods - all |
| Black tea | Honey | Vinegar |
| Blue Cheese | Milk | Yeast extract |
| Bread | Mushrooms | |

**Helpful Substances**

| | |
|---|---|
| Acidophilus | Olive oil (2tsp per day) |
| Citricidal | Garlic Capsules (plus eating lots garlic) |
| Live yogurt | |

**Note**

Be wary, when the Candida is being expelled from the system, it makes the person crave sweet things (which of course feed it, and keeps it alive). It is important that the Candida is killed off, otherwise the symptoms only get worse. I believe that Candida, out of control, leads to more acute problems, like ME.

# Foods in Balance

For a healthy mind and body, we need more alkaline than acidic foods in our system. An imbalance can create various digestive problems, skin rashes, and an assortment of other complaints, such as headaches, aches and pains around joints and the spine. It can also affect our mind and emotions. Too much acid could cause irritability, anger or frustration.

We would not consider filling up our petrol tank with the wrong kind of fuel and expect our car to run smoothly, but we will often put the wrong kind of food into our body without a second thought, and wonder why we do not feel so good.

We may listen to the adverts on the television, and could be subtly influenced by what appears to be a health-producing product. We must realise that the manufacturer is aiming to sell the product, so will tempt us in whichever way possible. Some of these "so called" healthy options may contain far too much acid, and may not be good for us.

As you will notice from the list below, oranges and orange juice are extremely acidic. We are led to believe that oranges, and their juice, are healthy, and contain lots of vitamin C. Oranges are shipped here from the country in which they are grown, and they may be picked under-ripe to minimise rot on the journey. When the fruit is under-ripe, it does not have as much vitamin C and contains too much acid. Often, vitamin C powder is added after it is juiced. Because of the acid content, we may suffer from irritable bowel, or aches in our muscles.

In my experience, children who have drunk orange juice for its vitamin C content have often suffered from sore throats, a persistent cough, or maybe chest infections. Many children suffer from eczema. Often this has been healed, just by leaving out all fruit juice, although cow's produce is often the greater offender. Fruit juice certainly will affect the enamel on childrens' and adults' teeth.

## Acidic Foods

| | |
|---|---|
| Sugar | Wine |
| Fruit Juices | Wheat (breaks down into sugars) |
| Nuts | Egg Yolk |
| Red Meat | Onions |
| Oily Fish | Tomatoes |
| Shellfish | Strawberries |
| Tea | Rhubarb |
| Coffee | Dairy Produce |
| Chocolate | |

## Alkaline Foods

| | |
|---|---|
| Dried Fruits | Most Vegetables (except those mentioned above) |
| Lentils | Most Fruits  (except those mentioned above) |

A vegetarian diet with a good variety of grains and vegetables, beans and pulses, with fruits that are eaten in the way they are grown, meaning not juiced, puts you squarely on the way to an alkaline diet.

Fats and sugars are the enemies, plus too many wheat-based foods, which break down into sugars, but of course can be eaten in moderation.

I have noticed over the years, working with clients who have allergies, wheat comes up more and more as an allergic food. Modern constituents of wheat-based foodstuffs cause a lot of acidity in the body. This, in turn, leads to bloating, constipation and wind problems, and because this is turned into sugars, we have an abundance of obesity problems too.

Because of the proliferation of convenience and processed foods, most of us now eat our foods much too quickly. As the foods are soft, we do not chew enough. This in turn stops our foods from getting digested properly. So, again, we finish up with more acidity in our system than our body can cope with.

So, chewing thoroughly, eating less of the fatty, sugary foods, and more of the alkaline foods will help us all onto a healthier path.

This is a very complex and important subject, and goes far beyond the scope of this workbook to go into. Fortunately, there are many good books and other sources of reference out there on nutrition and health, and some which focus on specialist vegetarian, coeliac, wheat-free, dairy-free and other dietary requirements.

# Cleansing Diet

Every so often it is a good idea to have a few days of cleansing the body. I find that after the winter months of feeding myself with stodgy foods, I really enjoy this diet, and it seems to boost my energy levels too.

It is important not to do this diet if you have kidney disease, diabetes, or an eating disorder, and of course, if you are pregnant.

Sometimes you may get spots or blemishes appearing. You could also have a slight headache or maybe a coated tongue. These are signs that your body is detoxing. Try not to take painkillers as your liver has to work hard to process these, and it defeats the whole process.

Sometimes when we detox, we can feel slightly worse before we get better, so follow the diet for one day, and the following day have an all-fruit or all-vegetable day, avoiding dairy and grains.

| | |
|---|---|
| **When You Wake** | Do some simple stretching exercises and take some deep breaths with the window open. Drink a large tumbler of filtered water with a squeeze of fresh lemon juice, or a couple of teaspoons of cider vinegar. Eat a kiwi fruit. |
| **Breakfast** | 12 fl.oz cranberry juice and mineral water (half water-half juice). Eat half a melon sprinkled with 1oz sunflower and pumpkin seeds. |
| **Mid-Morning** | 12 fl.oz filtered water and two bananas, which should be chewed well. |
| **Lunch** | 1 glass additive-free vegetable juice, making sure it is salt free (check the label) Eat half an avocado dressed with 1tsp olive oil and cider vinegar. |
| **Mid-Afternoon** | 12 fl oz grape juice and mineral water (half water-half juice). Eat 1 bunch of grapes. |
| **Evening Meal** | 12 fl oz filtered water, and eat as much fruit as you like, but not citrus fruit. |
| **One Hour Before Bed** | 1 small tub of live yogurt mixed with a little dried fruit. |

It is important not to do any heavy lifting whilst doing the diet, so resting and doing some simple exercise like walking in the fresh air would be good. Having an early night would be beneficial too.

# Helpful Foodstuffs and Remedies

ALOE VERA — Taken as a health drink in the morning with a little fruit juice. Good for energy, digestion, ulcers, constipation. For burns and scalds, keep an Aloe Vera plant in your kitchen, and if you do burn or cut yourself, break a small piece of the fleshy plant and gently dab the Aloe juice on the wound. It cools and helps the body to heal with no scarring. All kinds of cuts, wounds and skin rashes can also be helped by putting on Aloe Vera juice.

ARNICA — Homeopathic remedy for bruises, sprains and muscle aches.

ARSON ALB — Homeopathic remedy for anxiety and fear, food poisoning, and cramps in the legs.

BURDOCK ROOT — Anti-inflammatory, anti-bacteria/fungal. Liver cleanse. Good for boils, septic states and fevers.

CIDER VINEGAR — One of my favourite remedies. 1 tbsp in hot water first thing in the morning. It cleanses the system. There are so many areas in which cider vinegar can be used, so buying a book on the topic could be of great help to you. Not only for the body, but also around the home.

CAMOMILE TEA — A relaxing and calming tea, that is beneficial at bedtime with a spoonful of honey. Promotes a relaxing sleep.

CLOVES — Bruising cloves and steeping them in some hot water in which honey has been added is a soothing temporary toothache aid.

ECHINACEA — Taken when colds and flu are around. It boosts the immune system.

GOLDEN SEAL ROOT — This also boosts the immune system.

GINGER — Stimulates blood circulation, and is antiseptic.

GRAPEFRUIT SEED EXTRACT — Anti Candida, anti-worm/parasite.

LAVENDER OIL — Relaxant, good for burns, helps sleep.

LINSEED — Good for the colon, and particularly for diverticulitis.

MILK THISTLE — For digestion, anti-toxic, anti-inflammatory.

PEPPERMINT — Digestion, respiratory system and circulation.

BACH FLOWER RESCUE REMEDY — Carry around in your pocket for emergencies, or shock. The cream version soothes sore skin.

SEA-SALT — Use this in cooking instead of Table Salt.

SEA WEED — Adds flavour to many foods. Rich in iron and iodine. If you grow your own vegetables, look out for seaweed fertiliser from the garden centre. Putting this on your home grown veggies will produce iron-rich plants. Many types can be bought from health food shops.

SLIPPERY ELM — Very soothing, and protects intestinal walls from acid and toxins. Helps to heal ulcers and inflammation.

LECITHIN GRANULES — Helps reduce cholesterol. 3tsps/day on cereal or in yogurt.

# Vitamins and Minerals

| | |
|---|---|
| VITAMIN A | Guards against heart disease and strokes, lowers cholesterol levels and helps to slow down the ageing process. It enhances immunity and protects against colds, flu and infections. It also acts as an antioxidant, helping to protect cells against diseases and is necessary for new cell growth. A deficiency of Vitamin A can cause dry hair and skin dryness, and dryness of the eye. A deficiency includes skin disorders, including acne, weight loss. Beta-carotene is the best source of Vitamin A. Best natural sources are fish liver oil, liver, carrots, green and yellow vegetables, eggs, milk and dairy products, margarine, and yellow fruits. |
| BIOFLAVONOIDS | Often referred to as Vitamin P, this is essential for the absorption of Vitamin C, and should be taken together. Good for bruising, helps with the lowering of cholesterol levels. |
| FOLIC ACID | Good for the red blood cells, and is said to help depression and anxiety. Folic acid is very important in pregnancy, as it is vital for the developing baby and maybe prevent premature birth. Folic acid works best when combined with Vitamin 12 and Vitamin C. |
| PABA | A member of the B-complex family. Helps maintain a healthy intestinal flora and assists in the formation of red blood cells. If you have greying hair, brought on by stress, it is said that it can restore the hair to its original colour. It can reduce inflammation in arthritis, leading to more flexibility. |
| VITAMIN B COMPLEX | A mixture of the B vitamins, which help the nerves, skin, eyes, hair and liver. It can be helpful in cases of depression and anxiety. Some people who have been diagnosed with Alzeimer's have shown to be deficient in some of the B vitamins. |
| VITAMIN B1 | Good for the circulation, assists in blood formation, and the production of hydrochloric acid, which is important for proper digestion. Good for brain functions, and has a positive affect on energy, and acts as an antioxidant. Best natural sources of B1 are dried yeast, rice husks, whole wheat, oatmeal, peanuts, pork and most vegetables, bran and milk. |
| VITAMIN B5 | Helpful in treating depression and anxiety. Often called the anti-stress vitamin. It helps to convert fats, carbohydrates and proteins into energy. A deficiency may be seen as fatigue, with headaches. |
| VITAMIN B6 | For both physical and mental health. It can help in reducing symptoms of pre-menstrual syndrome. It is useful for treating allergies, arthritis and asthma. Properly assimilates protein and fat, reduces night cramps, and works as a natural diuretic. Carpal tunnel syndrome has been linked to a deficiency of Vitamin B6. Best natural sources of B6 are brewers yeast, wheat bran, wheat germ, liver, kidney, heart, blackstrap molasses, milk, egg, and beef. |

| | |
|---|---|
| VITAMIN B12 | Known as the red vitamin as it helps to prevent anaemia in regulating the formation of red blood cells helping to utilise iron. Good for digestion and the absorption of foods. Older people with memory loss and perhaps depression can be helped with Vitamin B12, as well as people who are vegetarians. B12 is not easily absorbed by the stomach, so a time release tablet would be more acceptable. Best natural sources are liver, beef, pork, eggs, milk and cheese. |
| VITAMIN B15 | Good for the immune system, helps in maintaining a high energy level. It can also help in reducing high blood cholesterol. It helps to extend the life of cells, protects against pollutants, protects the liver. Best natural sources are brewers yeast, whole brown rice, whole grains, and seeds. |
| VITAMIN C | An antioxidant, which helps tissue growth and repair. It helps with stress, and protects against infection and enhances immunity. Valuable if taken when colds are on the horizon. Acts as a natural laxative. Best natural sources are citrus fruits, berries, green leafy vegetables, tomatoes, cauliflower, potatoes, as well as sweet potatoes. |
| VITAMIN D | The 'sunshine vitamin', it helps with the absorption of calcium and phosphorus. It is important for the growth and development of bones and teeth. Taken with Vitamins A and C it can aid in preventing colds. Best natural sources are fish liver oils, sardines, herring, salmon, tuna, milk and dairy products. |
| VITAMIN E | An antioxident. It improves circulation and is useful in treating pre-menstrual syndrome. It can help reduce high blood pressure. Could help with infertility in men and women, and help with menstrual problems. Helps prevent and dissolve blood clots. Best natural sources are wheat germ, soya beans, vegetable oils, broccoli, and other green leafy vegetables, whole grains and eggs. |
| CALCIUM | For bones, teeth, and gums. Helps to regulate heartbeat. A deficiency of calcium can lead to aching joints, rheumatoid arthritis, brittle nails, high cholesterol and blood pressure, nervy disposition. Dolomite, which is a mixture of calcium and magnesium is better tolerated. Best natural sources are dairy products, soyabeans, sardines, salmon, peanuts, walnuts, sunflower seeds, dried beans, green vegetables. |
| CHROMIUM | Best taken as a chelated form of chromium, such as chromium picolinate. It helps by burning fat in the body, increases lean muscle, helps to speed up the metabolism and reduce sugar cravings. Chromium is needed for energy and is vital in the synthesis of cholesterol, fats and proteins. It also maintains stable blood sugar levels. Best natural sources are meat, shellfish, chicken, corn oil, brewers yeast. |
| IRON | We need iron for the red blood cells. Good for the immune system and for energy. Iron deficiency symptoms include anaemia, dizziness, fatigue, nervousness, obesity and slowed mental reactions. Taking iron in a tablet that is food based is |

|  | more easily accepted, and does not cause constipation. Best natural sources are red meats, dried fruits, eggs, nuts, beans, molasses, oatmeal. |

MAGNESIUM | Assists in calcium and potassium uptake. Helps prevent calcium deposits, kidney and gallstones. Magnesium can help prevent depression, dizziness, muscle weakness and twitching, pre-menstrual syndrome and also maintains the body's proper pH balance and body temperature. Promotes a healthy cardiovascular system. Dolomite contains Calcium and Magnesium, and is in perfect balance for the body to use. Best natural sources are figs, lemons, grapefruit, yellow corn, almonds, nuts, seeds, dark green vegetables, apples.

MANGANESE | Needed for healthy skin, bone and cartilage. Nuts, seeds, wheat germ, wheat bran, green leafy vegetables, tea and pineapple are all good sources of manganese.

POTASSIUM | Helpful for the nervous system and regular heart rhythm. It aids muscle contraction and works with sodium to control the body's water balance. Signs of deficiency include abnormally dry skin, constipation, acne, chills, depression, diarrhoea, nervousness, high cholesterol, insomnia, muscle fatigue and low blood sugar. It helps to dispose of the body's waste matter. Best natural sources are citrus fruits, watercress and all green leafy vegetables, mint leaves, sunflower seeds, bananas, potatoes.

SELENIUM | An antioxidant, especially when combined with vitamins A, C, E and Zinc. It protects the immune system by preventing the formation of free radicals that can damage the body. Selenium and Vitamin E act synergistically to aid the production of antibodies and to help maintain a healthy heart and liver.

ZINC | Important for a healthy immune system and wound healing. Very important for prostate gland functions and the growth of reproductive organs. Take zinc if starting a cold. A deficiency may result in a loss of taste and smell, and thinning fingernails that show white spots. Essential for protein synthesis, governs the contractibility of muscles, helps in the formation of insulin. Good for maintaining the balance of acid-alkaline fluids in the system.

# Healthy Living Tips

- Get up earlier in summer and later in winter, in rhythm with natural sunlight hours. Do not eat before you are fully awake.

- Eat when you are hungry, not out of habit. Graze rather than gorge. Eat little and often, with plenty of fruit snacks in between.

- Eat a mainly vegan diet, with half your intake of food consisting of fruit, vegetables, seed sprouts, nuts and seeds. If you wish to eat meat, avoid the intensively-reared kind. Choose fish or organic game instead. Eat these foods only with vegetables.

- Eat food as raw and unprocessed as possible. Avoid synthetic chemicals.

- Avoid concentrated foods such as sugar and sweeteners. Dilute fruit juices if you must have them. Drink at least 4 pints of water per day.

- Minimise your intake of dairy foods, and refined wheat and grains.

- Take frequent exercise, ideally in green, leafy places and natural countryside.

- If you are taking supplements, make sure that you are also taking a multi-vitamin and mineral supplement.

- Wash fruits and vegetables thoroughly – many gallons of pesticides have been sprayed on them.

- If you are drinking bottles of water, make sure that it is in a glass bottle and not plastic.

- Carbonated water depletes our minerals. People who consume large quantities of carbonated drinks will tend to have less density in their bones. Filtering and distilling water not only removes the pesticides and other impurities, but also removes the valuable minerals. You may need to supplement with added minerals.

- Buy organic foods whenever possible, preferably not grown in other countries. Better to grow a few vegetables and fruits for yourself.

- Do not use plastics or film on foods.

- Avoid alcohol, tea and coffee, as these cause the body to lose water.

- Fibre is obtained from whole-foods e.g. grains, lentils, beans, nuts, seeds, fresh fruit and vegetables.

- Make sure that you chew your foods thoroughly.

- Most of us eat too much saturated fat, but eating the right kind of fat is good for us. Essential fats reduce the risks of cancer, heart disease, allergies, arthritis, eczema, depression, fatigue, infections, PMS.

- Fats that heal : hemp, flax, soy-beans, walnuts, seaweed, sunflower seeds, sesame seeds, almonds, wild fowl, venison, chicken, fresh mechanically pressed oils in opaque containers, Evening Primrose oil.

- Fats that don't heal : eggs, butter, lamb, beef, some fish, roasted nuts and seeds, dairy products, pork, refined oils, margarines and shortenings.

- The Omega 6 fat family is linoleic acid, which the body converts into gamma-linoleic acid (GLA). Evening Primrose Oil and Borage Oil are the richest known sources of GLA. These oils keep the blood thin, which prevents clots and blockages, relaxes the blood vessels, lowers blood pressure, helps to maintain the water balance within the body, decreases inflammation and pain, improves nerve and immune function and helps insulin work, assisting blood sugar balance.

# Some Ingredients To Avoid In Personal Care Products

It is always a good idea to read the labels on all products, whether it be foods or toiletries. We may often study ingredients on food labels, but fail to see that such items as face creams, lotions shampoos and conditioners etc. may have damaging ingredients too. Everything we put on the skin gets absorbed by the body, just as if we had eaten it. So something that we put on the body may also make us ill. It is useful to check out the ingredients used in toiletries that we apply to our body, in case they could be having a damaging effect on us over a period of time :

| | |
|---|---|
| Propylene Glycol | Called a humectant in cosmetics, this is really industrial antifreeze and the major ingredient in brake and hydraulic fluid. Tests show it can be a strong skin irritant. Information about Propylene warns users to avoid skin contact as it can cause liver abnormalities and kidney damage. |
| Sodium Lauryl Sulfate | Sodium Laureth Sulfate (SLS) is used in testing laboratories as the standard ingredient to irritate skin. Industrial uses of SLS include garage floor cleaners, engine degreasers, and car wash soaps, just to name a few.<br><br>Studies show its danger potential to be great when used in personal-care products. One study indicates that SLS is systemic, and can penetrate, and be retained, in the eye, brain, heart, liver etc, with potentially harmful long-term effects. It could retard healing, cause cataracts in adults, and can keep childrens' eyes from developing properly.<br><br>Other research has shown that SLS and SLES may cause potentially carcinogenic nitrates and dioxins to form in shampoos and cleansers by reacting with commonly used ingredients found in many products. Large amounts of nitrates may enter the blood system from just one shampooing. |
| SLES | This is the alcohol form (ethoxylated) of SLS. It is slightly less irritating but may cause more drying. Both SLS and SLES can enter the bloodstream. They are used in personal-care products because they are cheap. A small amount generates a large amount of foam, and when salt is added it thickens to give the illusion of being thick and concentrated. |
| Petroleum | Same properties as Baby Oil. Industrially it is used as a grease component. Not easily absorbed by the skin. |
| Bentonite or Kaolin | Clays used in skin foundations that may clog and suffocate the skin. |
| Glycerin | Draws moisture from inside the skin and holds it on the surface for a better feel. Dries skin from the inside out. |

| Collagen and Elastin of High-Molecular Weight | Derived from animal skins and ground up chicken feet. Both of these ingredients form films that may suffocate and over moisturise the skin. |
|---|---|
| Bar Soaps | Made from animal fat that may let bacteria feed and grow in it. May corrode the skin and dry out. |

Many of the ingredients like collagen, elastin, and hyaluronic acids found in many cosmetics cannot penetrate the skin because their particulate size is larger than the pores of the skin.

# Common Environmental Chemicals

**FORMALDEHYDE ......**

Aerosol sprays
Air fresheners
Antibiotics
Antiperspirants
Antiseptics
Butter
Cavity wall insulation
Cements
Cheese

Milk products
Moth proofing
Mouth washes
Nail polish
Newspaper & newsprint
Orthopaedic casts
Paper manufacture
Permanent-press treatment
Petrol

Chipboard flooring
Concrete
Detergents
Diesel fuel
Disinfectants
Dyes
Fabric conditioners
Fertilisers
Foam-backed carpets & curtains
Foam rubber

Photography & photographs
Pillows
Plaster
Shampoo
Shrink-proofing
Smog
Soap
Soft plastics
Stretch fabric
Synthetic resins

Furniture
Glue
Hair setting lotion
Insecticides
Kitchen units
Manufacture of Vitamins  A & E
Matches
Mattresses
Mildew proofing

Tanning of animal skins
Toothpaste
Traffic fumes
Wall board
Waste incineration
Water – repellent treatment
Wood preservatives
Wood veneer
Wrinkle-resisting treatment

**HYDROCARBONS ......**

Air fresheners
Coal fires
Coal-tar soap
Cleaning fluids
Cosmetics
Deodorants
Detergents
Disinfectants
Heating oil
Lighter fuel
Liquid paraffin
North sea and Propane gas

Ointments
Paints
Perfumes
Petrol & diesel fumes
Polishes
Propellants in aerosol sprays
Solvents
Sponge rubber
Varnishes
Vaseline
Wax candles

## PHENOL ......

| | |
|---|---|
| Antiseptics | Nylon |
| Aspirin & other drugs | Plastics |
| Bakelite | Pesticides |
| Carbolic | Petrol |
| Cosmetics | Photographic solutions |
| Dyes | Polyurethane |
| Electrical insulation & wiring | Preservatives in medicine |
| Epoxy resins | Preservatives in pharmaceutical injections |
| Fireworks | Perfumes |
| Hard moulded plastics | Synthetic detergents |
| Hair dye | Sun screens |
| Herbicides | Skin lightener |

When we look at these lists, it really shows just how much we are being bombarded with chemicals in our lives. It is completely impossible to avoid most of these, but knowing what we may be sensitive to, and going for safer products is all going to help us to remain healthy and active.

## Tooth Amalgam

Over many years of working with Allergies, I have found that a high percentage of clients have tested positive for a sensitivity to Mercury and Amalgam. In the early days of my work, I was chatting to my dentist about this and he just laughed and said it was completely rubbish, as otherwise the dental association that he belonged to would have written papers about the side-effects. I asked him if he would let me have a small sample of Amalgam for testing, which he reluctantly gave me.

Over a period of time, at each visit to my dentist he sarcastically asked me how many people I had found to be allergic to Amalgam. It was on one of these visits that I noticed his attitude had changed. He said that he had just returned from a dental conference, and one of the lectures was centred around research that had been done on some side-effects regarding Amalgam. Tooth Amalgam had been put into the teeth of sheep, and the sheep all aborted their lambs. It was not long after this that he told me that he had to have special filters on his equipment fitted, to stop Amalgam going into the drains, when his patients were rinsing their mouths.

One of my clients came to me suffering from symptoms that included deep depression, lack of energy and feeling so ill that she had seriously considered suicide. On testing for allergies, I found that Tooth Amalgam was very high on the list. She said that she had a lot of this metal in her mouth, which was very worrying. She talked about the possibility of having these fillings taken out, but of course, it needed to be done safely, as when the metal is removed, some of the debris will be swallowed and get into the body's system. So after the consultation she researched for a dentist that would be able to remove the fillings.

I saw this lady about six months after she had gone through her treatment with the dentist, and I could not believe how well she looked. She no longer felt tired and depressed and certainly did not feel suicidal any more. I was delighted with her progress, and so pleased to hear that she was going to start her own business, something she would not have tackled before. Shortly after her visit she gave me a paper which her dentist had given her (see below).

## SELECTED HEALTH SYMPTOM ANALYSIS OF 1569 PATIENTS WHO ELIMINATED MERCURY-CONTAINING DENTAL FILLINGS

The following represents a partial statistical symptom summary of 1569 patients who participated in six different studies evaluating the health effects of replacing mercury-containing dental fillings with non-mercury containing dental fillings. The data was derived from the following studies: 762 Patient Adverse Reaction Reports submitted to the FDA by the individual patients; 519 patients in Sweden reported on by Mats Hanson, Ph.D; 100 patients in Denmark performed by Henrik Lichtenberg, D.D.S; 80 patients in Canada performed by Pierre Larose, D.D.S; 86 patients in Colorado reported on by Robert L.Siblerud, O.D.,M.S., as partial fulfillment of a Ph.D requirement and 22 patients reported on by Alfred V.Zamm, M.D., FACA, FACP. The combined total of all patients participating in the six studies was 1569.

| Symptom | Number Reporting | As % | No Cured or Improved | As % |
|---|---|---|---|---|
| ALLERGY | 221 | 14 | 196 | 89 |
| ANXIETY | 86 | 5 | 80 | 93 |
| BAD TEMPER | 81 | 5 | 68 | 89 |
| BLOATING | 88 | 6 | 70 | 88 |
| BLOOD PRESSURE PROBLEMS | 99 | 6 | 53 | 54 |
| CHEST PAINS | 79 | 5 | 69 | 87 |
| DEPRESSION | 347 | 22 | 315 | 91 |
| DIZZINESS | 343 | 22 | 301 | 88 |
| FATIGUE | 705 | 45 | 603 | 86 |
| GASTRO-INTESTINAL PROBLEMS | 231 | 15 | 192 | 83 |
| GUM PROBLEMS | 129 | 8 | 121 | 94 |
| HEADACHES | 531 | 34 | 460 | 87 |
| MIGRAINE | 45 | 3 | 39 | 87 |
| INSOMNIA | 187 | 12 | 146 | 78 |
| IRREGULAR HEARTBEAT | 159 | 10 | 139 | 87 |
| IRRITABILITY | 132 | 8 | 119 | 90 |
| LACK OF CONCENTRATION | 270 | 17 | 216 | 80 |
| LACK OF ENERGY | 91 | 6 | 88 | 97 |
| MEMORY LOSS | 265 | 17 | 193 | 73 |
| METALLIC TASTE | 260 | 17 | 247 | 95 |
| MULTIPLE SCLEROSIS | 113 | 7 | 86 | 76 |
| MUSCLE TREMOR | 126 | 8 | 104 | 83 |
| NERVOUSNESS | 158 | 10 | 131 | 83 |
| NUMBNESS ANYWHERE | 118 | 8 | 97 | 82 |
| SKIN PROBLEMS | 310 | 20 | 251 | 81 |
| SORE THROAT | 149 | 9 | 128 | 86 |
| TACHYCARDIA | 97 | 6 | 68 | 70 |
| THYROID PROBLEMS | 56 | 4 | 44 | 79 |
| ULCERS / SORES IN ORAL CAVITY | 189 | 12 | 162 | 86 |
| URINARY TRACT PROBLEMS | 115 | 7 | 87 | 76 |
| VISION PROBLEMS | 462 | 29 | 289 | 63 |

# Working with the Spine

Unless you are an Osteopath or a Chiropractor, you should not attempt to adjust the spine. The reason for including this exercise is that we could be suffering from all kinds of ailments, and not even think that it could be associated with the spine being out of alignment.

I always check out the spine when I am treating my clients, and by dowsing down the chart, I ask the question "is this vertebrae perfectly aligned". If the answer is "No" then I mark the chart, and continue to the bottom. I mark other vertebrae in the same way. I then check the symptoms associated with the vertebrae(s) in question, and usually they tie up with the symptoms my client is experiencing.

As I am not a Chiropractor or an Osteopath, I send my client off to have an adjustment with one of the above professionals, if I find there is a need. I am always interested to see what adjustments were made, as it is good to have some confirmation of what I have found as being misaligned in the spine.

The Spine is like a central pole that holds up the body, with muscles and tendons supporting it. The spine consists of 24 vertebrae, or small bones. There are 7 vertebrae in the neck, which are called cervical, 12 in the upper back called thoracic, and 5 in the lower back called lumber. There are also 5 fused bones that form a continuation of the spine, called the coccyx.

Each vertebra has a hole running through it, which houses the spinal cord. Attached to the spinal cord are the roots of the nerves, which link them to the brain. These nerves if damaged, can cause much discomfort and pain, or even paralysis. The spine can be damaged in many ways, which can cause pain and immobility. Lifting heavy objects, sitting badly, or even sleeping on a bed that is not as supportive as it should, can all cause the spine to malfunction.

Tough bands of fibre hold together the spinal joints, and the vertebrae are protected by fibre discs, which are shock absorbers. Each joint is surrounded by strong muscles that get their messages from the brain, which makes the muscle contract. This in turn causes the various joints to move as required.

Exercise, good posture and drinking plenty of water help the spine to stay supple. In Acupuncture terms, the Bladder Meridian runs from the inner corners of the eyes, over the head, down the neck, into the back, and into the legs, finishing up at the small toes. It is one of the longest Meridians, and will affect the functioning of the spine if we are dehydrated, so drinking plenty of water is important.

## The Spine and Chakras

The spine is not only important for supporting our physical body, but it is also very important for our spiritual enlightenment. Yoga teaches that there are a series of subtle energy centres situated along the spinal column. These are called Chakras, which really mean 'wheels' because they spin. These are connected together by nerve channels that run down each side of the spinal column. Each Chakra has its own sphere of influence, which can be listed as follows:

1. At the base of the spine, in the region of the coccyx
2. Just below the navel
3. Solar Plexus
4. Heart Centre
5. Throat
6. Between the eyebrows
7. Crown

At the base of the spine is the home of that mysterious power known as 'Kundalini'. The word itself means 'coiled up' and refers to the belief that the Kundalini power lies coiled like a snake in its home, and is said to be the latent spiritual force in man, which when aroused,

| Area Supplied by Nerve | Results of Nerve Impingement |
|---|---|
| **1C** Blood supply to the head, the pituitary gland, the scalp, bones of the face, the brain itself, inner and middle ear, the sympathetic nervous system | **1C** Headaches, nervousness, insomnia, head colds, high blood pressure, migraine headaches, mental conditions, nervous breakdowns, amnesia, epilepsy, infantile paralysis, sleepng sickness, chronic tiredness, dizziness or vertigo, St, Vitus Dance |
| **2C** Eyes, optic nerve, auditory nerve, sinuses, mastoid bones, tongue, forehead | **2C** Sinus trouble, allergies, crossed eyes, deafness, erysipilas, eye troubles, earache, fainting spells, certain cases of blindness |
| **3C** Cheeks, outer ear, face bones, teeth, trifacial nerve | **3C** Neuralgia, neuritis, acre, pimples, eczema |
| **4C** Nose, lips, mouth, eustachian tube | **4C** Hay fever, rose fever etc., catarrh, hard of hearing, adenoids |
| **5C** Vocal cords, neck glands, pharynx | **5C** Laryngitis, hoarseness, throat conditions like a sore throat, quinsy etc |
| **6C** Neck muscles, shoulders, tonsils | **6C** Stiff neck, pain in upper arm, tonsillitis, whooping cough, croup |
| **7C** Thyroid gland, bursa in the shoulders, elbows | **7C** Bursitis, colds, thyroid conditions, goiter |
| **1D** Arms from the elbow down, including the hands, wrists and fingers, esophagus, trachea | **1D** Asthma, cough, difficult breathing, shortness of breath, pain in lower arms and hands |
| **2D** Heart including its valves, and covering, also coronary arteries | **2D** Functional heart conditions and certain chest pains |
| **3D** Lungs, bronchial tubes, pleura, chest, breast, nipples | **3D** Bronchitis, pleurisy, pneumonia, congestion, influenza, grippe |
| **4D** Gall bladder, common duct | **4D** Gall bladder conditions, jaundice, shingles |
| **5D** Liver, solar plexus, blood | **5D** Liver conditions, fevers, low blood pressure, anemia, poor circulation, arthritis |
| **6D** Stomach | **6D** Stomach troubles including nervous stomach, indigestion, heartburn, dyspepsia etc |
| **7D** Pancreas, islands of Langerhans, duodenum | **7D** Diabetes, ulcers, gastritis |
| **8D** Spleen, diaphragm | **8D** Stomach troubles, hiccoughs |
| **9D** Adrenals or super-renals | **9D** Allergies, hives |
| **10D** Kidneys | **10D** Kidney troubles, hardening of the arteries, chronic tiredness, nephritis, pyelitis |
| **11D** Kidneys, uterers, | **11D** Skin conditions e.g. acne, pimples, eczema, boils etc., auto-intoxication |
| **12D** Small intestines, fallopian tubes, lymph circulation | **12D** Rheumatism, gas pains, certain types of sterility |
| **1L** Large intestines or colon, inguinal rings | **1L** Constipation, colitis, dysentery, diarrhea, ruptures or hernias |
| **2L** Appendix, abdomen, upper leg, caescum | **2L** Appendicitis, cramps, difficult breathing, acidosis, varicose veins |
| **3L** Sex organs, ovaries or testicles, uterus, bladder, knee | **3L** Bladder troubles, many knee pains |
| **4L** Prostate gland, muscles of the lower back, sciatic nerve | **4L** Sciatica, lumbago, difficult or painful or too frequent urination, backaches |
| **5L** Lower leg, ankle, feet, toes, arches | **5L** Poor circulation in the legs, swollen ankles, weak ankles and arches, cold feet, weakness in the legs, leg cramps |
| **S** Hip bones, buttocks | **S** Sacroiliac condition, spinal curvatures |
| **C** Rectum, anus | **C** Hemorrhoids or piles, pruritus or itching, pain at end of spine when sitting |

enables man to achieve a state of ecstasy. This is said to occur when the Kundalini, having been awakened, rises up the nerve channels of the spine, pierces the Chakras, and finally reaches the Crown Chakra, situated in the cortical area of the brain.

When the Kundalini energy reaches this area, true bliss is achieved. It is the state of super-consciousness, and it is from this centre, when in a calm and meditative state, we become masters of our destiny, and we become one with the universe.

# The Importance Of The Chakras

Chakras are pulsing wheels of light that draw in energy to the vital organs of the body. These wheels correspond with the endocrine glands, which sends hormones into the body. Colours are also associated with these areas. There are many books written on this subject, giving detailed information, so seeking these may be helpful.

When we are born, we are very much linked in with our mother's energy system, and we share her aura for a while. As we begin to grow and develop, we open up to our own Chakra system and take on our own aura.

## BASE CHAKRA (RED)

Affects us between birth and the age of seven. This is situated at the base of the spine and is related to the physical body.

So, as the baby develops into childhood, this Chakra begins to open up and comes into flower. It is associated with the 'physical', so we find that the baby is very active with movements, such as walking, running, jumping, and generally being very physical.

## SACRAL CHAKRA (ORANGE)

Affects us between seven and fourteen. The sacrum is our creative area, or productive area. Between seven and fourteen this Chakra begins to develop and flower.

As it suggests, this is the area where the sexual organs are situated. It is a time when we begin to physically change. Girls breasts develop and they begin to have regular periods, preparing them for motherhood when the time comes. Boys' voices deepen, and boys and girls become more aware of each other as opposites. As this is a creative area, we may often find that creative gifts, like drawing, painting, making things, or anything artistic may start to develop as the Chakra opens.

## SOLAR PLEXUS CHAKRA (YELLOW)

Affects us between fourteen and twenty-one. This is when we start to think about what we want to do with our life. We may have developed hobbies and interests and could be stretching ourselves on a mental level. We may find ourselves preparing for our future with learning and job choices, often testing ourselves out in some way or other.

This is when the Solar Plexus Chakra comes into action. This area is often called the anxiety area (the home of butterflies when we feel scared). It is a time for finding out who we are, and testing out our strengths and weaknesses. We are searching for our path. Adrenals and Pancreas can be affected by stress or anxiety.

## HEART CHAKRA (GREEN)

Affects us around twenty-eight. Around twenty-eight to thirty we can be a bit more settled in life. Maybe we are now in a satisfying career, or in a firm relationship. There could be a family at this time. Note that this Chakra lines up with the outstretched arms, and is the place where we draw others into our heart, and trusting that others will accept us into their heart also. So it is about giving and receiving. This will affect us in all aspects of life, whether it is a fulfilling job, or family life.

## THYMUS CHAKRA (PINK)

This area is very much associated with the green Heart Centre. When we feel loved and accepted for who we are, we learn to love ourselves. This is a very important Chakra, for if we do not love ourselves, and do not feel loved and accepted by others, we constantly bend over backwards

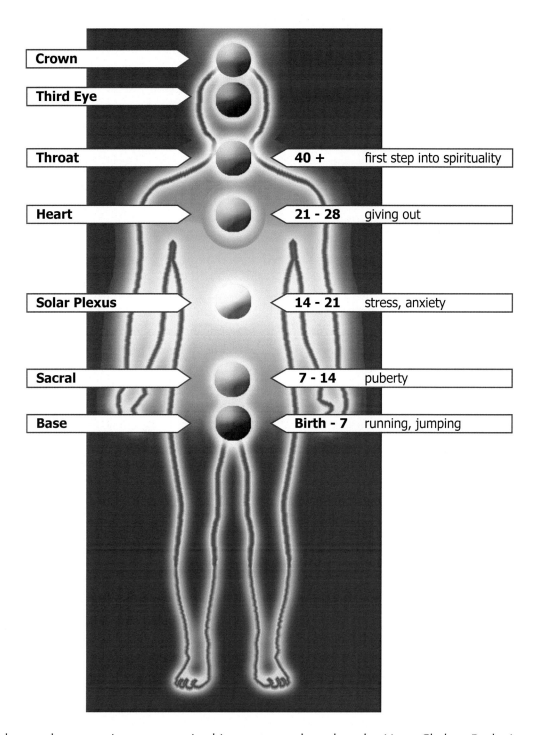

Crown

Third Eye

Throat — 40 + — first step into spirituality

Heart — 21 - 28 — giving out

Solar Plexus — 14 - 21 — stress, anxiety

Sacral — 7 - 14 — puberty

Base — Birth - 7 — running, jumping

to please others, causing us to strain this energy, and weaken the Heart Chakra. By loving ourselves, we give this area balance.

People who work as healers or therapists should be aware that they must love themselves by taking care of themselves. So it is most important that they seek treatments or rest for themselves, to strengthen this area. Beware of what my husband used to call 'the greed of giving.'

## THROAT CHAKRA   (PALE BLUE or TURQUOISE)

Around forty to fifty we should be able to free ourselves up from the physical. Although we still need our body, our aim is now towards Spirituality. It is a place where we have learnt from past experiences, and have gained much wisdom over the years.

This is the place when we speak our truth, we know who we are and know where we want to go. We can help others with this wisdom, and others may seek us out for this wisdom.

## THIRD EYE CHAKRA   (INDIGO)

Located between the eyebrows, this Chakra is the area of intuition. When we allow mind to relax, and we switch off to everyday activity, we can tune into the Third Eye area, and get in touch with our Higher Consciousness. This helps us to deal with the burdens of everyday life. We can use the power of thought to help us to achieve perfection as we see it to be.

The Sanskrit name is Ajna, meaning 'to know' or 'command'. By meditation, or visualisation we can achieve our highest goals. A person becomes what they believe they can be, from knowing. Success comes from knowing you have done your very best.

## CROWN CHAKRA   (VIOLET)

Located at the top of the head, it is the seat of the highest frequency of energy. Often depicted in  pictures of saints as having a halo around the head. As we journey through all of the Chakras starting with the Base, we grow and develop. We arrive at the Crown, where we can reach a state of extreme bliss, union with the Source, one with all of Nature.

Although I have given ages for these Chakras to flower, we can develop at differing ages. I am sure we have all known young people that seem to have reached wisdom and spirituality far beyond their years. In the same way, we can also find older people who really do not seem to have worked through the lower Chakra system.

Sometimes, younger people may have experienced sexual abuse. When this has happened, energy from the Base Chakra surges through the other Chakras, possibly damaging them. The same can also happen when people might experiment with drugs and alcohol at an early age.

# Balancing the Chakras Through Dowsing

The stresses and tensions of life can cause a Chakra to be out of balance, as well as leading to negative thinking and actions. When we become affected by these, the Chakras do not spin in the way they should, so vital energy is not taken into the body. This means that organs in the area of the Chakra become sluggish.

For example, when we worry a lot, or are not speaking up for ourselves, the throat Chakra could be out of balance. As a result, we could suffer from stiff neck, sore throats, maybe stumbling over words in a conversation, or even having a tickly cough that is difficult to heal.

The following dowsing exercise, performed every so often, is helpful in keeping the body in balance :

- Firstly, we need to discover a 'healing finger.' If you usually dowse with your right hand, the healing finger will be on the left hand. If you usually dowse with your left hand, the healing finger will be on the right hand.

  Dowse over each of the fingers on that hand asking *"Is this my healing finger ?"* There will be one finger that will come up with a positive signal. Once you have discovered that finger, you will be ready to work.

- Dowse over the Chakra diagram, and ask to be shown which, if any, of the Chakras are out of balance. There could be more than one. If you find that you have several out of balance, dowse again to see in which order they need to be balanced. For instance, if there are three to be balanced :

  - put your finger on one Chakra and ask *"Is this the first chakra to be balanced?"* If *"No"* then check the others, putting your finger on each and asking *"Is this the first chakra to be balanced"* until you have identified which one it is.

  - Repeat this process now, asking *"Is this the second chakra to be balanced?"*
  - Continue with the third, until you get the correct order.

- Now, sit down quietly, and imagine your Crown Chakra opening up, then visualise energy pouring down through the Crown Chakra, then Third Eye Chakra, through the Throat Centre, along the shoulder, down the arm, and pouring into your healing finger, which will be placed on the first chakra to be healed.

  As you do this, set the pendulum in a circular movement. The pendulum will change direction when the healing has come to a stop.

  If there are other chakras to heal, repeat the same process until all have become balanced.

  When you have finished, check again *"Are all my chakras balanced now?"* If not, repeat the process.

# The Bach Flower Remedies

The list below is just an abbreviated version of what the remedy is about. A worthwhile book to buy is "Bach Flower Therapy" by Mechthild Scheffer. Published by Thorsons.

| | | |
|---|---|---|
| 1. | Agrimony | For those who do not show their true face to the world |
| 2. | Aspen | Secret fears |
| 3. | Beech | Critical, arrogance, intolerance |
| 4. | Centaury | The doormat, easily exploited |
| 5. | Cerato | Lack of confidence in own decisions |
| 6. | Cherry Plum | Fear of loss of control. Uncontrolled temper |
| 7. | Chestnut Bud | Repeats same mistakes over and over again |
| 8. | Chicory | Manipulating, interfering, conditional love |
| 9. | Clematis | The daydreamer |
| 10. | Crab Apple | The perfectionist. Feels unclean, stuck in detail |
| 11. | Elm | Weak moments in the life of strong people |
| 12. | Gentian | Easily discouraged. Refusing to be guided |
| 13. | Gorse | Oh what's the use attitude. Despair |
| 14. | Heather | The needy child |
| 15. | Holly | Jealousy, distrusts, fears that one is deceived |
| 16. | Honeysuckle | Constantly referring to the past, not here now |
| 17. | Hornbeam | Monday morning feeling. Mental exhaustion |
| 18. | Impatiens | Impatient, irritable. Too much of a hurry |
| 19. | Larch | Insecurity. Expects to fail |
| 20. | Mimulus | Known fears |
| 21. | Mustard | Periods of deep gloom. Soul in mourning |
| 22. | Oak | The struggling, exhausted fighter |
| 23. | Olive | Exhaustion after strain or illness |
| 24. | Pine | Guilt, despondency |
| 25. | Red Chestnut | The over-caring person |
| 26. | Rock Rose | Terror, panic, acute states of fear |
| 27. | Rock Water | For those who are very hard on themselves |
| 28. | Scleranthus | About poise and balance. Lost direction |
| 29. | Star of Bethlehem | For shock, re-orientation. Awakenings |
| 30. | Sweet Chestnut | Dejection, isolation, abandoned |
| 31. | Vervain | Highly strung, fanatical, wants 150% achievement |
| 32. | Vine | Dominating, striving for power. Ambitious |
| 33. | Walnut | New beginnings, fresh start |
| 34. | Water Violet | Isolation, reserved, will not burden others |
| 35. | White Chestnut | Unwanted thoughts going around in head |
| 36. | Wild Oat | No ambition. Lost direction. Bored |
| 37. | Wild Rose | Apathy, lack of interest. No motivation |
| 38. | Willow | Bitterness. *"Poor me"* attitude |
| | Rescue Remedy | For emergencies. Comforts, calms. A mixture of Cherry Plum, Clematis, Impatiens, Rock Rose, Star of Bethlehem. |

# Using the Bach Flower Remedies

In the 1980s, a friend and I travelled to the Bach Flower Centre in Wallingford, Oxon. We were attending a weekend course on learning about the Bach Flower Remedies. Unfortunately, on our journey to the Centre, we found ourselves completely lost, and spent a frazzled couple of hours, asking directions, and losing ourselves again. When we finally arrived, we were not in good shape, as we both were feeling hot and very tired by our ordeal.

I remember walking up the driveway to the house, and suddenly feeling as if I had entered another world. It was just like slipping back in time. There was an extraordinary feeling of peace and tranquillity everywhere. Looking at my friend's face I could see that she also was affected by the atmosphere. Neither of us spoke, but we just looked at each other and smiled. I knew that this was going to be an enriching weekend for us both.

I shall never forget that weekend. The presence of Dr Bach was everywhere, and to actually see the flowers that were used in the preparations, growing in such a tiny garden. We were shown around the Doctor's house, which was extremely simple. He had made much of the furniture himself, and it really looked as if he had just popped out for a few minutes even though he had died peacefully in his sleep in 1926.

Dr Bach was a physician, homeopath, Harley Street specialist, consultant and a bacteriologist. He began his career as a medical student at Birmingham University, and qualified in 1912. When treating his patients, he became more interested in their moods and emotions, than their diseases. He studied the way in which they behaved. Those that had a cheerful outlook made better progress. Those that lacked hope, or were unhappy did not do so well.

He began to see disease as an end product of unhappiness, fear or worry. He wondered what could be done to restore peace and harmony and because he was intuitive, he knew there would be an answer within nature.

Dr Bach gave up his practice in Harley Street in 1920 to study plants and flowers all over the English and Welsh countryside. As he was very intuitive, he seemed to be led to the correct remedies, and the more he worked with the plants, the more sensitive he became. This resulted in him taking on some of the negative symptoms of the flowers, and he experienced great terror and extreme mental torture. Sometimes he would be in an intense state of anguish until the right remedy was found to relieve his suffering.

He started using the remedies on his patients with great success, and moved to the Thames Valley in 1934, near Wallingford, which is where the Bach Centre is to this day. At the age of 50, Dr Bach died peacefully in his sleep, not long after he had completed the last of his 38 remedies. In a lecture he said :

> *"The action of these remedies is to raise our vibrations and open up our channels for the reception of the Spiritual Self; to flood our natures with the particular virtue we need, and wash out from us the fault that is causing the harm.*
>
> *They are able, like beautiful music or any glorious uplifting thing, which gives us inspiration, to raise our very natures, and bring us nearer to our souls and by that very act, bring us peace and relieve our sufferings.*
>
> *They cure, not by attacking disease, but by flooding our bodies with the beautiful vibrations of our Higher Nature, in the presence of which, disease melts away as snow in the sunshine.*
>
> *There is no true healing unless there is a change in outlook, peace of mind, and inner happiness."*

Dr Bach did not want his flower remedies to be used only by the medical profession; they were simple enough to be used by lay people. Both my friend and I left that weekend filled with a desire to carry on the work of Dr Bach. I had used the remedies before, but I felt I had a better understanding of where they came from now. I had dabbled with other types of flower remedies, but always came back to the Bach Flowers for some reason.

I felt a little apprehensive, as the Centre had told us that the way that we discover what remedies are needed for our client is by counselling, and by listening to what was going on in that person's life, and treating accordingly. I could see that would work, but in my experience, I have found that clients often kept a lot to themselves. I said that I would use dowsing to find the remedies, and was immediately told that this was not acceptable. In fact, they went as far as to ask me to sign a paper promising that I would never use dowsing to find the remedies. I said that I could not do this, and so they refused to issue me with my certificate.

I felt quite unhappy about this, and did not use the flower remedies for quite awhile. It was not until I started to get the programme together for 'Emotional Stress Release' that I just knew the flower remedies would be perfect for healing after the negative emotions were released. And so I did dowse, and was amazed at how accurate they were in detecting the areas needing to be healed. I felt sure that Dr Bach would approve of this quick and simple method of using his remedies, and so from that day on, I used dowsing to detect the remedies. Dr Bach was intuitive, and I am sure he would have dowsed if he had known about it. The Bach Flower Centre, I know, want to keep everything just as Dr Bach used the remedies, and I respect them for that, but I think, for me, I have to use the remedies in the way that I have found they work best, and dowsing for them has proved to be extremely successful.

Dosage:
- 2 drops of each of the chosen remedy in 30ml Winchester bottle with a pipette.
- Add 6 drops of brandy or apple cider vinegar to keep fresh, fill the bottle with water and shake well.
- Dowse to see how long the remedy needs to be taken.
- When finished, dowse to see whether another remedy(s) should be taken.

The remedies do not always need to be taken internally, as they can be put on the skin, or used in the bath. Everyone can benefit from the remedies, very young, very old, animals and even your plants.

At some time or other, we all will benefit from a remedy. Life is a journey, and sometimes we fall. The remedies are the 'helping hand' to lift us back on the road to recovery.

I had a client telephone me and ask whether I treated animals. I said that I did not really, but what was the problem. My client said that she had a new cat, and it was terrified if anyone came to the door, like the postman or dustman or if there was any other noise, the cat flew behind the fridge. I said that I thought that Mimulus would be a good remedy, which is for known fears. I left my client to buy the remedy, and promptly forgot all about it. Two weeks later my client rang me and she said that the remedy had worked fantastically. In fact, did I have a remedy now for a brazen cat, that wanted to take over the whole household ! We laughed, and I left her dowsing for the next remedy.

# The Twelve New Era Tissue Salts

At home, I have a cupboard full of helpful remedies for when they may be needed, either for myself or for one of my family. The New Era Tissue Salts are the remedies that I mostly use because I find that these are the ones that seem to be most effective. They are so simple to use, and as the pills are small and quick to dissolve, they can be given safely to young children.

## What Are The New Era Tissue Salts ?

The New Era Tissue salts are minerals, no different to the earth's rocks and soil. They are the building bricks of the body and make up the body's bone, blood, organs and muscles.

In the 19th century Dr. Schuessla discovered that when a human cell was reduced to ashes, it contained all of the twelve Tissue Salts. The Tissue Salts are present in foods, particularly when they are grown in an organic way. By developing the Tissue Salts, Dr. Schuessla discovered that if there was a deficiency of a particular Tissue Salt in the body, certain symptoms were experienced. By taking a particular Tissue Salt, the body returned to normal. Of course, the New Era Tissue Salts should not take the place of any medication that your doctor has prescribed.

The remedies are numbered 1 to 12, and you will notice that if you were born under a certain sign of the Zodiac, you could find that this will highlight a certain area where you may have a need for a particular Tissue Salt.

| REMEDY NO 1. | CALC. FLUOR (Calcium Fluoride) |
|---|---|
| Description | Found in the surface layer of bones and teeth. Also in the connective tissue. It helps to tone. |
| Deficiency Symptoms | Enlargement of blood vessels, varicose and enlarged veins, or weakening of abdominal walls. Abscesses with hard hard callous edges or hard, knotty protuberances on bone surface. |
| Astrological Sign | CANCER   (Earth Mother) |
| Note : | May also need Silica |

| REMEDY NO.2 | CALC. PHOS (Calcium Phosphate) |
|---|---|
| Description | The most abundant salt in the body and definitely needed for proper growth and nutrition as it strengthens bones and helps build new blood cells. Particularly helpful to the elderly because of its restorative power after acute diseases. |
| Deficiency Symptoms | Bone diseases, slow healing fractures, defective nutrition, poor teeth, coldness, cramp, chilblains, colds, catarrh. Subjects needing Calc Phos are often helped by warm sunny weather. |
| Astrological Sign | CAPRICORN   (Mystical) |

| REMEDY NO.3 | CALC. SULPH (Calcium Sulphate) |
|---|---|
| Description | In the body this mineral occurs in connective tissue, as blood constituent and also in the liver cells. The function in the latter is the removal of worn out blood cells from the circulation. |
| Deficiency Symptoms | Late destruction of cells, producing lesions, inflammation and pus. Pimples, skin eruptions, frontal headaches, liver and kidney upsets. |
| Astrological Sign | SCORPIO   (Positive, determined people. Can be sarcastic) |

**REMEDY NO.4**      **FERR. PHOS (Iron Phosphate)**

Description

Oxygen transporter. Found mainly in the red blood corpuscles and helpful for the first stage of all inflammation, wounds due to injuries, and haemorrhages. Nose bleeds.

Deficiency Symptoms

Anaemia. Relaxation of muscle fibres

Astrological Sign

PISCES (Artistic, imaginative)

**REMEDY NO. 5**      **KALI. MUR (Potassium Chloride)**

Description

Good for childhood diseases. Found in the blood, the muscles, nerve and brain cells as well as the intercellular fluid. Blood tonic.

Deficiency Symptoms

Acute inflammations. Coating of the tongue. Glandular swellings. Discharge from mucous surfaces. Scaling of the skin.

Astrological Sign

GEMINI (Curious)

**REMEDY NO. 6**      **KALI. PHOS (Potassium Phosphate)**

Description

Found in all fluids and tissues, notably brain, nerve, muscle and blood cells. Tranquilliser.

Deficiency Symptoms

Anxiety, fear, depression, neuralgia, nervous exhaustion, or prostration. Atrophy in old people. Intense odour.

Astrological Sign

ARIES (Rules the head, mental activity)

Note

Also may need CALC FLUOR

**REMEDY NO.7**      **KALI. SULPH (Potassium Sulphate)**

Description

An oxygen carrier of special significance to the skin like eczema. Supports liver functions.

Deficiency Symptoms

Deposit on the tongue. Discharge of watery secretion from mucous surfaces. Helps the third stage of inflammation.

Astrological Sign

VIRGO (Solar plexus. Active and ready to learn. Could be critical)

**REMEDY NO.8**      **MAG. PHOS (Magnesium Phosphate)**

Description

Part of muscles, nerves, bones, brain, spine, teeth, and blood.

Deficiency Symptoms

Cramps, spasms and pain often accompanied by exhaustion and sweat. Constipation in infants, headaches, toothache, colic.

Astrological Sign

LEO (Needs to let go and relax)

**REMEDY NO. 9**      **NAT. MUR (Sodium Chloride)**

Description

Found in every liquid and solid of the body. Regulates the degree of moisture within the cells.

Deficiency Symptoms

Bloating due to water retention in the intercellular fluid. Drowsiness, chill, tearfulness, and salt cravings. Loss of taste/smell. Hay fever, constipation, eczema, gum ulcers, runny nose.

Astrological Sign

AQUARIUS (Studious and thoughtful)

**REMEDY NO.10**   **NAT. PHOS  (Sodium Phosphate)**

Description
Found in blood, muscles, nerve and brain cells as well as in intercellular fluid, productive in catalysing lactic acid and emulsifying fatty acids.

Deficiency Symptoms
Poor digestion of fats. Thin, moist coating on the tongue and yellowish creamy-look soft palate. Diarrhoea, spasms, pains and fever. Acidity.

Astrological Sign
LIBRA  (Drawn to justice or legal work)

**REMEDY NO.11**   **NAT. SULPH  (Sodium Sulphate)**

Description
Found in the intercellular fluid where it helps to eliminate water.

Deficiency Symptoms
Poor digestion. Water retention. Yellow watery secretions on the skin. Excessive bile, causing such things as coating at the base of the tongue. May put on weight easily. Engorged lymph system. These people need encouragement and affection.

Astrological Sign
TAURUS  (Patient, plodding and determined)

**REMEDY NO.12**   **SILICA  (Silicon Dioxide)**

Description
Found more in plants than animals. However, essential to the body in bones, joints, glands, skin and mucous surfaces.

Deficiency Symptoms
Malnutrition, bone aches, chronic pus formation, chronic rheumatic conditions. Pimples, spots, styes, boils. Patients requiring this may suffer from cold feet. May have bad memory. This remedy could help those in advancing years.

Astrological Sign
SAGITTARIUS  (Jovial, bright and generous. May exaggerate)

**CALC SILICA**

Description
This affects most organs in the body where dehydration has been an ongoing problem for possibly many years, and the information pathways around the body have been compromised.

# Absent Healing

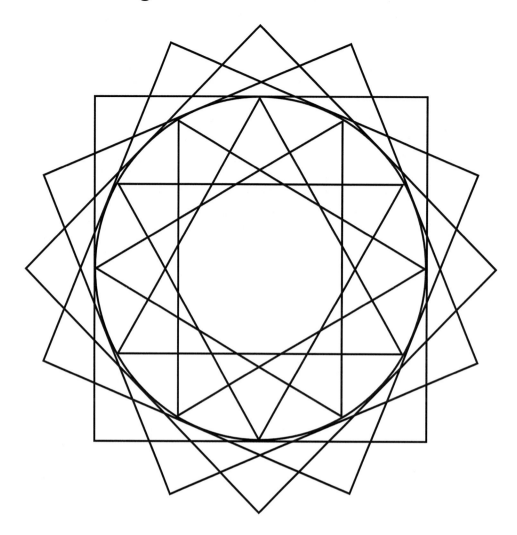

Using this diagram to send absent healing to someone is a very simple but an effective process. Remembering, firstly, to ask :

> *"May I work with this person?"*
> *"Should I do this?"*
> *"Can I do this?"*

and getting positive responses to all, then proceed.

So that you can focus fully on that person, write his/her name on a small piece of paper, such as a 'Post It Note' and place it in the centre of the diagram. Keep your mind completely on that person as you set the pendulum in the healing mode.

Circle the diagram with the pendulum, and visualise your Crown Chakra opening up and Spiritual Energy pouring down from the Crown into your Third Eye Chakra, then your Throat Chakra, down into your Heart Chakra. From there, the Spiritual Energy goes across to your arm, and down into the hand that is holding the pendulum. So now, as the pendulum swings over the person's name, healing takes place. Stay in this position, with the pendulum swinging in a circular manner, until it naturally slows down.

When the pendulum has stopped moving, dowse to see whether you need to send a Bach Flower remedy, or a tissue salt, or a colour to that person. If the answer is *"Yes"* to these questions, dowse to see which remedy, salt or colour needs to be sent, and put the remedy on the diagram. For example, if it is a colour, mark the 'Post It Note' with the colour chosen, using a felt tip pen. Dowse to see how long you need to leave the remedy there, and also whether you need to send more healing at another time.

A few years ago, Mrs. M, a client who usually came to see me on a regular basis, cancelled an appointment just before she was due to arrive. She had a bowel problem, and found, just as she was about to leave to attend her appointment with me, she had to rush to the toilet urgently, leaving her in a lot of pain and unable to drive. She was very apologetic but made a new appointment for the following week. Because I now had an hour before my next client arrived, I decided to send Mrs. M some absent healing. I did all the things I have stated above, and let the pendulum swing for about 10 minutes. On her next visit, my client said she had felt very guilty about cancelling the last appointment with me, as a short time after she had she put the telephone down after speaking to me, she had felt so much better, in fact much better than she had felt for a while. I told her what I had been doing, and she said she had definitely felt something happen.

Another lady, who was an author, came to me with a high level of stress. She wrote novels for a well-known publishing company. She had a large number of books to her name, and was well thought of. She explained that she was being sued by another writer for taking his ideas, which she emphatically denied. It was all getting quite nasty. After giving her support in other dowsing ways, I suggested that we do some absent healing. She looked quite shocked, because healing this man was probably the last thing she wanted to do. When I explained that I was going to send absent healing, to heal the situation, it made much more sense to her. So we set up the healing diagram, and asked *"May I?" "Should I?" "Can I?"* in the usual way, which all came up as very positive. She wrote his name on the 'Post It Note' and together we did the healing circle with the pendulum as before. At the end of the healing, I dowsed and found that healing needed to be sent at a certain time over the next few days. I promised her that I would do this for her, and she promised to let me know if there was any change in the situation. I did this, and really forgot about the situation. It is not often that I read the newspapers, as they are often full of negative information. However, a client had left a newspaper behind after a treatment, and I picked it up and was about to throw it out when an article caught my attention. It stated that 'A well known author had dropped the case against another author that he was suing'. I had a phone call later that day from the lady, saying things had got back to normal for her now, and how pleased she was.

These case histories are only two brief examples of the healings that have taken place over the years, but there are many, many more where peoples' lives have been changed in some way. The absent healing method is very simple, but very powerful.

# Clearing Negative Energy from Property

## Clearing Negative Earth Lines

Draw a rough diagram of the property. This does not need to be to scale. Mark in the names of the dining room, living room, toilet, bathrooms, etc. Dowse over the whole of the diagram, and ask :

> *"Are there any negative earth lines in this building or surrounding land?"*

If the answer is *"Yes"* dowse over each of the rooms on your diagram to find out where this negative energy is, perhaps marking the area with a cross. There could be several places. Then, tune into the building, and say :

> *"I want to clear any negative energy from this building and surrounding land"*
> *"Can I do it?"*
> *"May I?"* and
> *"Am I ready to do it now?"*

If *"Yes"* is your answer to all of these questions, proceed. Using your imagination, think of a snowy white sheet, and imagine that this snowy white sheet is passing right under the property, and it is gently being pulled up into a 'swag bag' by spiritual beings. This swag bag is encasing the whole of the building and land surrounding. Imagine that this is now being transferred to a spiritual compost heap to be recycled into something positive.

Dowse to check that the task has been successfully completed.

## Clearing Negative Psychic Energy

Dowse over the whole of the diagram again and ask :

> *"Are there any entities in this building, or surrounding land?"*
> *"Are they having a negative effect?"*

Sometimes the answer to this second question will be *"No"*, because that entity needs to be there for some reason or other. They are not all bad. However, if the answer to this second question is *"Yes"*, dowse to see where the entity/s is/are, and mark on your diagram.  State what you want to do :

> *"I want to remove any entities from this building and surrounding land"*
> *"Can I do it?"*
> *"May I do it?"*
> *"Am I ready to do it now?"*

 If the answers to these questions is *"Yes"*, stand in the place that needs to be cleared, and say :

> *"It is now time to move on, you have been trapped here for a long time.  I am going to help you meet up with your friends and family on the other side. They have been waiting to welcome you for a long time. You are forgiven for any wrongdoing. You are free to move on. I will now give you a column of light (visualise this). Step inside this column of light."*

As you visualise a column of light, say out loud, or in your head :

> *"May all thought forms, any soul fragments, traumatic events, memories and restless spirits now move into this column of light for safe transition, and be transmuted and transformed, each to it's appointed place. In peace and love ......* So be it.*"*

Now, light a candle and sprinkle sea salt around in the area you have cleared. Check to see that this has been cleared.

Sometimes this process may need to be repeated. If so, when does this need to be done - 1 week? 1 month? 6 months? Dowse for an answer.

*Insanity - doing the same thing over and over again
and expecting different results.*

Albert Einstein

## II. Emotional

When we look at emotions, we realise that there are many levels to them. On the surface we can have a smiling face, but underneath we could be experiencing self-doubt, fear, anxiety, and similar feelings. The smile on our face is like a mask that we wear, so that nobody can see who we really are. The feelings underneath are very real though, and affect us in a number of ways. When we access these feeling during the following exercises, there is a great relief, and we may shed a few tears, or in some cases, laugh in an hysterical way, but this is good, as its a way of letting go, and helps us to move on to being a stronger person, without needing the mask.

I was speaking to a friend recently, and she was saying how she blamed herself so many times when things went wrong, she thought that she should know better, she really felt that she should know all the answers. All the things that happen in our life are things that we should be learning from, but we will not have all the right answers, and that is part of the journey and the learning. If these things did not happen, and we were all the same, we would all be like Barbie Dolls. We laughed at the end of our conversation, when I passed on a phrase that my husband used to say, which was *"So what?"*

So, when things are not going as you think they should try a *"So what."*

# Emotional Stress Release

When I started using dowsing for healing the body, running dowsing courses, and seemingly getting very good results, I realised that perhaps this was possibly the way that I could heal emotions. I could see that I had hang-ups from the past that showed up from time to time, and so had other members of my family. So I started experimenting with different ways of clearing the debris from the past. Eventually I came up with something that seemed to work beautifully. I practised on myself and my family, and was amazed to find that the method even cleared blocks from the womb and past life.

So, on my next dowsing course, I asked the participants whether they would be interested in working with the emotions. The response was overwhelmingly positive, and so I ran my first course in teaching this method. I was delighted with the way in which it went, and the feedback from the day was wonderful. I must admit that we all dipped into the paper tissues a lot on that day, and Rescue Remedy was dripped onto the tongue often. Even though we dug out a lot of negative stuff, peoples' faces were smiling as well as tearful. They all admitted that the day had been emotional, but they felt lighter, and that was quite evident.

So teaching Emotional Stress Release was now part of my courses, and each time I could see that things had moved on. It was later that I decided that Spirituality would complement the other two days and this became Part 3 of my course.

I must say that my large family have been very interested in what I have been doing over the last few years, so much so that I have children and grandchildren who now use my methods of dowsing for healing, and we have all seen and felt the benefits of this way of healing.

I have been delighted to discover that my eldest son Mark has developed the Emotional Stress Release to include Ancestry, and so, with his permission, I have included his technique in the Spiritual section. I am really looking forward to feedback from my former clients.

## How Clearing Works

Once we have helped the physical body to become healthier and more balanced, we are now ready to release our emotional blocks through dowsing. We can isolate and clear blockages from present time, as well as from the past. This enables us to move forward freely, helping us to reach our life's goals. It is possible to reach back and clear any blockages from pre-birth, and even baggage from Karmic experiences, helping us understand lessons that are to be learnt.

This might all sound too good to be true, but I have been using this method, not only for myself, but many others that come to me for treatment, or who have attended my courses, over many years. I never cease to be amazed at how such a simple treatment, has such astounding results. I have seen people change dramatically, even after one session, so I am eager for you to learn this technique too.

Think of the brain split into two. The left side is the logical side, and the right side is the emotional side. One side of the brain may contain a bad memory, or a fear or anxiety, whilst the other side can be very strong and resilient. There will be times when both sides of the brain will hang on to those memories, but these can be healed.

What we also need to understand is that signs and symbols have a huge effect on our mind and body. Think of the footballer, who thinks that if he puts on his 'lucky' socks, he will have a good game. How many people cross their fingers, if they wish for something good to happen. There are religious symbols that people wear. The sign of the cross. The waving of the flag. A lucky penny, and so on. So, using signs and symbols to clear emotional stress also works in the same way.

## Releasing Emotional Stress

So let us think of someone sitting in front of you who has emotional baggage to clear. Have a writing pad to hand, as well as your pendulum and the Feeling Words list (see page 68). When we dowse to see what feeling words we need to use, we are tuning into the person's subconscious, and their subconscious really wants the best for them, so we need to trust this process.

The first thing we do is to ask the age of that person at their next birthday. We do that because if we ask the age of that person, and their birthday was several months ago, we will miss out if something has happened during those last months since their last birthday. So, for instance, if the person you are working with is 25, you put down the age as in their 26th year.

Start by writing down their age. In our example that is - 26th year. Now dowse to see which year the emotion we are clearing is in. So ask :

> *"Is it in this person's 20th year?"*
> *"Is it in their 10th year?"*
> *"Is it in their 5th year?"*
> *etc.*

all the time dowsing until it comes up as a positive movement.

If it comes up at 5th year, also ask is it more than the 5th year. If it is a *"No"* it is the 5th year, and if it comes up *"Yes"*, ask if it is 6th or 7th, until you get a positive *"Yes"*.

Now we need to identify the emotion, or Feeling Word (see page 68), to clear from that year. We can dowse to find this word. I have split the list into columns and sections to make this process quicker.

So, first, running your finger down each column, ask :

> *"Is the Feeling Word in this column?"*
> *"Is it in this column?"*
> *"Is it in this column?"*

When you have identified the column, then dowse each of the sections in that column to see if the feeling word is in that section. Running your finger over the words in each section ask :

> *"Is the Feeling Word in this section?"*
> *"Or this section?"*
> *"Is it this section?"*

until you have narrowed the possibilities down. Then it is easier to individually dowse the few words in that small section to find the specific Feeling Word.

I have found that this is a better and quicker way to identify the word you need, than having to go down each of the words individually in all three columns.

So for instance, if you pick up that the person is in their 26th year, and that we need to look at the age of 7, and the feeling word associated with that age is ANGER, you are ready to help the person release this emotion. So this is the first part of the clearing. Now I will show you how to use symbols to clear this emotion.

- To integrate the two parts of the brain, where the memory is stored, ask your partner to extend their arms horizontally out to the sides with the palms facing forward. The left palm mirrors the left side of the brain, and the right palm mirrors the right side of the brain.

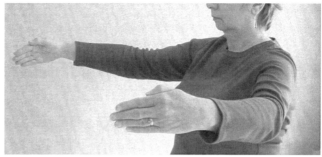

- Ask your partner to bring the palms together, linking the fingers, and at the same time to say:

    *"I release my anger from 7"*

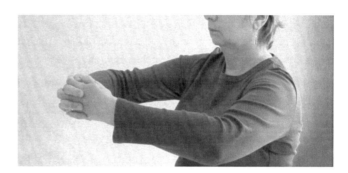

- Now bring the linked fingers into the heart, and again say :

    *"I release my anger from 7".*

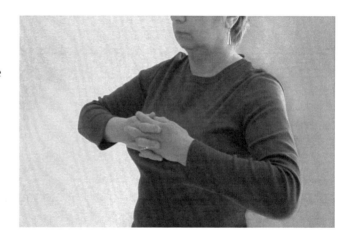

It is helpful if you do these actions with your partner, not only to give them confidence, but if you have an emotion in this area, you can clear it for yourself too. Then dowse to see whether this has cleared. In the majority of cases, it will have cleared, but if not we will use finger modes.

## Finger Modes

In Kinesiology, finger modes are used often. They relate to differing areas of the body. The finger modes, each touching at the finger tops, that we are going to use are :

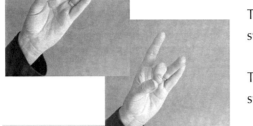

Thumb and index finger :
symbolising Muscle, Bone and Tissue.

Thumb and middle finger :
symbolising Nutrition, which includes food and oxygen.

Thumb and ring finger :
symbolising Emotions (this symbol comes up the most for clearing the emotions)

Thumb and little finger :
symbolising Electric Circuits. This relates to the electrical circuits, or meridians of the body, used by acupuncturists.

So, supposing when you checked whether this emotion of Anger had cleared, and it came up that this was not so, you will need to check through each of the fingers, to see which area needs to be used.

For instance, when you dowsed each of the fingers, let us say it came up positive on the Emotional finger. Get your partner to put their thumb and the emotional finger together, ask them to hold their arms in a horizontal position, with arms out to the side as before, and to say again, as they bring the fingers together :

*"I do release my anger from 7"*

now link the fingers together, and say again :

*"I do release my anger from 7"*

and then once more into the heart :

*"I do release my anger from 7"*

Check it out again to see whether it has cleared this time.

There maybe other areas to clear, from other ages, but when it comes up as nothing more to clear, an Affirmation needs to be said to help seal the healing of the emotions.

Check the list of Affirmations (see page 69) to see which one is right for your partner to say. Saying the Affirmation, and at the same time having the ring finger and thumb together and doing the movements as before helps the phrase to be accepted.

It is often helpful to say this also at bedtime, for a few days.

## Using Surrogates

I had the pleasure of a visit from my nephew and his wife recently. John was born deaf and his wife, Angela, is partially deaf. It is lovely to see them communicating with sign language, and lip reading. Angela told me that John gets quite frustrated when at work, as people do not know how to communicate, and often he is left alone and becomes isolated, which creates a lot of stress.

As I was testing them both for food allergies and what kind of supplements they might need, I asked if they would also like me to work with Emotional Stress Release. They both agreed, and we cleared several things for Angela, which was quite easy as she had partial hearing and could voice the words. When it was John's turn, I used Angela as a surrogate for him. Sitting close together, I asked Angela to put her foot close, and touching John's. As I found the ages and the feeling words to be released, Angela did the arm movements and voiced the words to clear the feelings. At the end, I wrote down the affirmation so that John could internally read for his homework.

Being a surrogate is being part of another person's energy field, and so responses made by one can be helpful to the other.

This is very helpful also when a mother brings a young child or a baby for allergy testing. Sometimes I pick up that there was stress at birth, or pre-birth, or there had been some kind of trauma in its short life. I get the mother to put the child on her lap, and as I pick up the feeling words, mother does the arm movements, and says the words. It is often lovely to see the little one trying to do the arm movements with mother, and I am often amazed at how the child quietens, and seems to tune into what we are doing.

People with a handicap of some kind can be helped enormously with Emotional Stress Release. So often, people with a disability carry a huge amount of stress, because of the way they have to adapt to life.

# Past Lives

I believe that we have lived many lives before we came into our present body. Each life is like a classroom where we learn skills, and begin to understand ourselves and others, and develop. As a small child in this lifetime, I have learnt skills, and adaptability, bringing me to here and now.

I may have made mistakes during this journey, but this is all about growing and developing. In the same way, we may have made mistakes in past lives, and maybe hurt ourself, or others. Sometimes we repeat the same mistakes over and over again. There is no punishment for this, but we do have to see what it is like being on the other side of a mistake - how it has affected others around us. So, if we have inflicted hurt onto someone in the past, often we have that kind of hurt placed on ourselves in another life, so that we can see the wisdom of both sides of the situation. We could be very timid in this lifetime, be too open to criticism, and display a poor self image. This could be due to abuse in a past life and wanting to please others. Sometimes the message is *"Please love me"* and so we try too much to please others so that they will love us, resulting in being the doormat for others.

When I discovered a way of clearing emotions from our past lives, by doing Stress Release, I found that I felt stronger and more balanced. I could tackle the everyday obstacles with a lot more confidence, and I felt a hidden strength that I had not experienced before. So if it was doing that for me, I certainly wanted this passed on to others.

Perhaps you do not believe that there are past lives. You could of course just skip over this section, or otherwise do the clearing as an exercise, without putting too much pressure on yourself about believing.

## Starting Off

As you have done before, ask the age of your partner at their next birthday. Let us say it will be their 26th year.

26. Dowse, going back in 10s, ask :

*"is the feeling to be released in this person's 26th year, 20th year, 10th year"*

until you get a positive response for the age that the feeling needs to be released.

If you are going back to a past life, you may need to clear something in this life first, before you get to the past.

When you have discovered the age where a feeling has to be cleared, dowse down the Feeling Words sheet to find the emotion to be released. Putting thumb and emotional finger together, repeat the arm movements as before saying :

*"I release my feelings of ............ from age ............"*

Check to see whether it has cleared. If not, you may need to use a different finger mode. If so, dowse to see which one it is, and repeat the arm movements again, saying :

*"I release my feelings of ............ from age ............"*

Clearing the emotions from this life, helps us to lead into another life. You will find, after working with this for a while, that the Feeling Words will be very similar to each other, and form a kind of pattern.

What eventually will happen, as you are dowsing and clearing blockages, is that it will go back to birth, and before birth. When you dowse, and the pendulum indicates that there is something to clear before birth, ask :

*"Is this in the womb ?"*

If the answer is *"Yes"*, ask whether it is conception :

*"1 month in the womb, 2 months in the womb ........ "*

and continue until you have found the right age again. Find the Feeling Word that you need to clear as before, and say :

*"I release my feeling of ............ at (which month) in the womb"*

until it has cleared.

Often a baby has many dangers to overcome in the womb. Sometimes mother's body may think that the baby is a foreign body, and try to remove it, in a threatened miscarriage. Mother may have problems herself, with worries and anxieties, and the baby may pick up on this. I often pick up that there is a lot of fear and terror around 7 months in the womb. Sometimes at this time, the placenta thinks it has finished its job and starts breaking down. It does need to do this at sometime nearer the birth, as this stimulates the baby to start preparing for birth. When it starts to break down earlier, it sends a lot of acid blood to the child instead of the nourishing food. This can be dangerous, or perhaps the child is in the wrong position for birth. So it is another world in the womb, and not always a cosy experience.

So going back to the dowsing again, if you dowse and it does not come up for anything to clear in the womb, then ask :

*"Is there something to clear from a past life?"*

If there is a positive swing for a *"Yes"*, proceed as follows.


**Past Life Issues**

Dowse to see which century you need to work in, starting at 21<sup>st</sup> 20<sup>th</sup> 19<sup>th</sup> etc. until you discover the right one. It does come up with BC from time to time.

- Ask whether this person was male or female?
- Are we looking at the way this person died?  eg. accident, sickness, killed.
- Did they die young?
- Were they a good person, or did they harm others?  (do not be afraid of this, as I said before, we all make mistakes)

When you have gone through a few more questions, to get a picture of what went on there, you can ask :

*"Is there anything else of importance that you need to know at this time?"*

Get a general picture about what went on, but not too deeply, as sometimes it is possible to take on the feelings from that time into the person's life now. Dowse for the feeling words again, and release as before, saying :

*"I release my ............ feelings from the ............ Century"*

using the finger modes as before.

Keep asking for any other feelings until it comes up that there is nothing more to clear. Make sure that you now find an Affirmation to seal you off from the past life.

Now come back to this life, and the age in which the person is now, and ask whether there is anything to clear from this age. If there is, clear in the usual way. Then find another Affirmation to finish off.

No more should be done on this for a few days, so that adjustments can be made to your memories.


# Clearing Miasms

A Miasm is a link or a thread that links us to our ancestors, and any disease or ailment that they may have experienced. All ancestors had some illness or other. It is not to say that you will inherit this disease, but because all things are passed through the genes, you may experience similar problems.

For instance, I know for a fact that way back in my family line, my ancestors suffered from tuberculosis, and in my family now, we often suffer from catarrh, chest colds, and allergy to cow's produce (tuberculosis was often passed on from cows into their unpasteurised milk). Some family members suffer from irritations like hay fever, or eczema.

By dowsing over each of the Miasms, find out whether any could be having an effect. You may find that you link in with more than one Miasm. By taking the Bach Flower Remedy prescribed for the Miasm, it halts the genetic link to your ancestors.

| Miasm | Bach Flower Remedy |
| --- | --- |
| Syphilis | Vervain / White Chestnut / Impatiens |
| Tuberculosis | Pine / Hornbeam |
| Psora | Holly / Scleranthus / Oak / Crab Apple |
| Conorrhoeal | Rock Rose / Cerato |
| Cancer | Star of Bethlehem / Pine |

When you have dowsed to see which Miasm you need to work with, put six drops of the remedy in a bottle, and fill up with filtered water and a small amount of brandy, or cider vinegar, to keep the remedy fresh.

Take six drops of the remedy, twice per day for six days. Dowse at the end of the six days to see whether it has cleared the Miasm.

If you need to work with another Miasm, dowse to see when you need to start that remedy (usually about one week) and repeat the process.

# Feeling Words

| | | |
|---|---|---|
| Abandoned | Haughty | Sorrow |
| Anger | Helpless | Stubborn |
| Aggressive | Hopeless | Stuck-up |
| Arrogant | Humiliation | Suppressed |
| Apprehensive | Hurt | Shock |
| Awful | Hurried | Smug |
| Argumentative | Impatient | Sad |
| Ashamed | Insecure | Shy |
| Anxious | Incapable | Stupid |
| Aggravated | Impossible | Scared |
| | | |
| Boredom | Injustice | Sceptical |
| Bitter | Irritated | Stifled |
| Blind | Intolerant | Spiteful |
| Brokenhearted | Inadequate | Terror |
| Burdened | Irresponsible | Torment |
| Betrayed | Imposed upon | Teased |
| Concerned | Indecisive | Troubled |
| Confused | Jealous | Too much responsibility |
| Criticised | Longing | Thoughtless |
| Claustrophobic | Lonely | Trauma |
| | | |
| Difficult | Left-out | Unaccepted |
| Disorganised | Lies | Undesirable |
| Defensive | Lost | Unneeded |
| Distressed | Let-down | Unfriendly |
| Depressed | Misunderstood | Uneasy |
| Doubt | Mean | Unfulfilled |
| Dirty | Miserable | Unpleasant |
| Deceived | Nauseated | Unhappy |
| Disappointment | Neglected | Unhelpful |
| Disloyal | Nervous | Unsuccessful |
| | | |
| Discontent | Obligated | Unwanted |
| Drained | Oppressed | Used |
| Discouraged | Overwhelmed | Unworthy |
| Disgusted | Paranoid | Useless |
| Egotistical | Punished | Unsociable |
| Embarrassed | Powerless | Unconcerned |
| Exasperated | Pain | Unloved |
| Envy | Pity | Unreliable |
| Empty | Pressured | Upset |
| Failure | Provoked | Unrespected |
| | | |
| Fear | Panic | Vindictive |
| Forced | Rejection | Wasted |
| Forlorn | Repulsive | Worthless |
| Forsaken | Resentful | Weary |
| Futile | Restless | Wrong |
| Frigid | Restriction | Wounded |
| Frustration | Selfish | |
| Grief | Shameful | |
| Guilt | Shattered | |
| Hate | Sour | |

# Affirmations

I love and respect myself
I let go of bitterness and blame
I now take up the path I am meant to follow
It is time to let go of the past
The only adult I need take care of is me
The past no longer affects me
I am strong and fulfilled
I cultivate a positive, hopeful outlook
I am at peace with myself
I have all the courage I need

I deserve to be happy
It is OK to trust my intuition
I no longer need to feel angry
I have hope and confidence in the future
My body is beautiful
Every day is a new day
I welcome the future
It is safe for me to grow up now
I have all the time I need
I give up all limiting notions

I can risk doing what is right
I am ready for excitement and adventure
Letting go is easy
It is now time to take charge of my life
I am gentle and good to myself
I am in charge of my life
I want to get well
I can stand up for myself
Every day I am stronger
I know what is right for me

I can do anything
I love myself just as I am
I am strong and energetic
I am master of my own fate
I let go of struggling so hard
I feel awake and fresh
I let go of guilt and shame
Calm flows through me
I radiate peace and calm
Hope brings healing

I am safe and secure
I am calm and courageous
I am enthusiastic about life
I learn from my mistakes
I deserve the very best in life
I am here now
I deserve  to get well
My feet are firmly on the ground
I enjoy being me
I have faith in life

I am ready for anything
I am secure within myself
I know what is right for me
I am a fortunate being with individual gifts
I think clearly and decide easily
I am ready for change
Every day is a new opportunity
I am calm and serene
I see things as they are
I have a strong sense of purpose
I am joining in

# The Ancestors

Many of our fears, anxieties and unexplained feelings are inherited from our ancestors. This may be the cause of us repeating old patterns over and over again. This of course stops us moving forward and being the person we are meant to be.

I am very lucky that many members of my family embrace what I teach, and use it for their own development, including several of my grandchildren. When my son Mark developed this part of the Stress Release technique, it was a great eye opener. As a family, we started using this method of clearing, and enormous changes began to take place. We all know when one of us is clearing some debris from the past, as we can all feel the changes, and we all move on.

Again, like before, this is a very simple process. Work with the Ancestors chart in this section to help you focus. What we are trying to do is identfy with whom there is an emotional block, what Feeling Word most closely represents that block, and then to clear that block, in order to enable us all to move on.

'Me' on the chart could be yourself, or you could use your client or partner's name in here. Firstly, dowse and ask the question :

*"Is there something to clear from the ancestors?"*

If the answer is a *"Yes"*, dowse over the names on the chart, perhaps putting your finger on each of the figures to help focus on each of the ancestors.  Start by asking :

*"Is the focus on the brother(s)?"*          *"Is the focus on the sister(s)?"*

If you get a *"Yes"* identify which brother/sister it is.  If *"No"* then ask :

*"Is the focus on the 'mothers' side?"*          *"Is the focus on the 'fathers' side?"*

You might get a *"Yes"* to one or both.  Let's say you get a *"Yes"* to the mother's side. Ask :

*"Is it the mother?"*

If the answer is 'No' go back a generation on the mother's side and, putting your finger on each figure, ask :

*"Is it the 'grandfather?"*          *"Is it the 'grandmother'?"*

If the answer is *"No"* go back another generation, and use the diagram to ask :

*"Is it this great grandfather?"*          *"Is it this great grandmother?'*

until you identify the root of the blockage with a positive swing of the pendulum. Now dowse for the Feeling Word associated with this person.  When you have identified this word, and, let's suppose the word was 'Angry' from one of the great-grandfathers on the 'Mothers' side, use the arm movements and finger modes as before, and say :

*"I release the angry feelings for my 'great grandfather'.*

Dowse to check that this has cleared, and then dowse to see whether there are any other feelings that need to be cleared from the 'great grandfather' until all has been cleared.

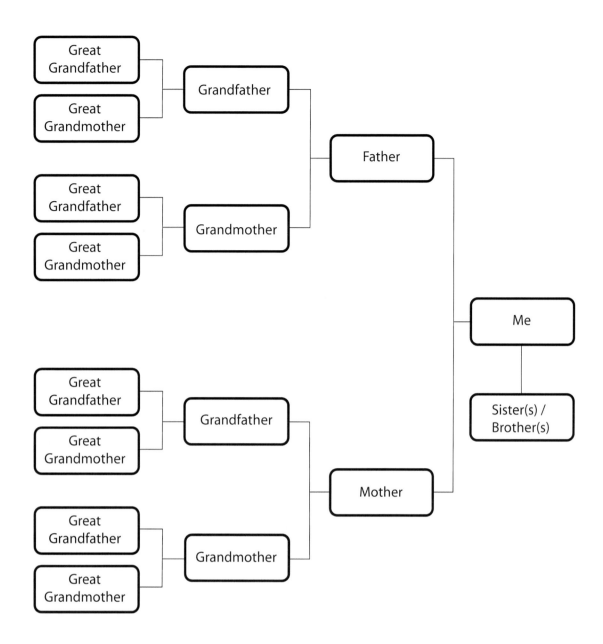

If, at the beginning, you got a *"Yes"* to the question *"Is the focus on the father's side"* too, then go back and repeat this process for the father's side through to its conclusion as above. When all is cleared, and after confirming that this is acceptable, then make this request :

" *I request permission to install an affirmation to my 'great grandfather.'*

Dowse for the answer. If this comes up as acceptable, use the arm movements as before, and say :

" *I command love and harmony into my ancestral family, and I clear these problems for future generations.*"

Then bring both hands into the chest and say :

*"It is done, it is done, it is done."*

Now check to see whether there are any personal emotions to clear for yourself, and finally find and use another Affirmation for yourself.

*Life is full and overflowing with the new.*
*But it is necessary to make room for the new to enter.*

Eileen Caddy

# III. Spiritual

This is the section where we can use colours, signs and symbols. When teaching this section as Part Three on my dowsing course, I love to see the look of surprise on faces as we work through some of these areas. It is often seen as a magical transformation, as it further opens the door to help and remove many more blockages.

As I used dowsing to help heal my clients, and teach my methods to others, 'Spiritual' just appeared at the right moment to complete the areas I am presenting now. I believe that there is a time and a place for everything, and when you reach this part of your learning, be confident that it is the right time for you also. Be prepared to be amazed by your results.

It is very important that you work through each of the sections in order. Working on the Physical side first, enables stability in the body, which prepares you for Emotional Stress Release. When you reach Spiritual, you should be balanced, and able to complete the last part of this teaching.

For this section you will need felt tipped pens in RED, ORANGE, YELLOW, GREEN, PINK, PALE BLUE, INDIGO, AND VIOLET. You will also need a dropper bottle that is about 30ml size.

# Colours

**RED Ray**

Characteristics

It has been called the great energiser, because it has a huge effect upon the physical body. Red is for heating - think of a lovely red fire. It warms up the blood in the arteries, which is good for the circulation. Red controls the Base Chakra, which is situated at the base of the spine, this in turn will affect the lower limbs.

Subjects prone to

Ailments of the bloodstream, which include anaemia, physical debility, colds, circulatory, and paralysis.

As a treatment

Stimulates the base Chakra, causing adrenalin, stored in the ductless glands, to be released into the bloodstream. So Red is therefore very useful in pushing us on to another level, taking us out of a sluggish situation.

Helpful foods

Beetroot, radishes, red cabbage, watercress, spinach, aubergine, red skinned fruits, black cherries, plums

**ORANGE Ray**

Characteristics

It stimulates the creative energy within the mind, and encourages us to reach higher for wisdom. Orange is warm and cheerful. It controls the Sacral Chakra, and affects the functions of the spleen by releasing worn out blood cells, and enabling the pancreas to be helped by releasing digestive juices.

Subjects prone to

Chronic asthma, phlegmatic fevers, bronchitis, wet cough, gout, chronic rheumatism.

As a treatment

Orange can help inflammation of the kidneys, gall stones, prolapse, and mental debility. Orange can have a freeing-up action upon body and mental functions. It is important that we do not over-stimulate with orange. We could become over-indulgent, so moderation with orange is to be recommended.

Helpful foods

Most orange-skinned vegetables and fruits, including carrots, swedes, pumpkins, oranges, apricots, mangoes, tangerines, peaches.

**YELLOW Ray**

Characteristics

Yellow has an alkalizing effect, which can strengthen the nerves. Yellow is also stimulating, and awakens the spirit, inspiring us to greater things. It gives us confidence, through opening the door to a higher mentality. Yellow also has an enriching effect upon the intellectual departments of the brain. Yellow stimulates the third Chakra, at the solar plexus level. The solar plexus houses many nerve endings controlling the nervous system. Some would call this area the abdominal brain. By becoming stronger and more confident, the third Chakra leads us on to understanding ourselves more, and seeking our true path. It also controls the digestive processes in the stomach.

| | |
|---|---|
| Subjects prone to | Stomach troubles, indigestion, constipation, flatulence, liver problems, diabetes, piles, eczema and skin problems. Nervous exhaustion would also fall into this category. |
| As a treatment | Yellow helps to cleanse and purify the system through the eliminative action of the liver and intestines. It can improve the texture of the skin by healing scars and other blemishes. |
| Helpful foods | Parsnips, yellow peppers, golden corn, yams, bananas, marrow, pineapple, lemons, grapefruit, melons, and most yellow-skinned fruits and vegetables. |

## GREEN Ray

| | |
|---|---|
| Characteristics | The wonderful vibrant green of fresh leaves in early spring is the most effective colour for healing. It gives us the courage to move on, giving us strength and balance. Green can sooth the nervous system, and calms the mind, which in turn can lower blood pressure. When we are in a calm state it can give us the confidence to bring others into our heart centre, and opens us up to loving others. In life we can become too self-centred, but by learning to share our love, we blossom. |
| Subjects prone to | Hearing troubles, blood pressure, ulcers. |
| As a treatment | Green is invaluable for helping to ease headaches and neuralgia. |
| Helpful foods | Most green vegetables and fruits. |

## BLUE Ray

| | |
|---|---|
| Characteristics | The calming effect of blue brings a feeling of tranquility. Again, like the effects of green, and its calming effect, a summer's day with a beautiful blue sky has a powerful effect on us. Blue affects the Throat Chakra. |
| Subjects prone to | All throat troubles, laryngitis, goitre, sore throat, hoarseness. |
| As a treatment: | Blue helps to control fever, high emotions, palpitations, vomiting, diarrhoea, inflammations, stings, and other forms of pain. |
| Helpful Foods | Most blue fruits, blue plums, bilberries, blueberries. |

## INDIGO Ray

| | |
|---|---|
| Characteristics | The Chakra is the Third Eye area, situated in the middle of the forehead, and controlling the pineal gland. It is our internal eye, whereby we can internally visualise our sense of direction. In my belief, it is also the area that most of us use when healing, or when using dowsing. So this area is extremely powerful, enabling us to grow and develop spiritually. |
| Subjects prone to | Eye troubles, ear and nose complaints, and other facial complaints. Indigo can often help with lung problems too. |
| As a treatment | Indigo is a purifier of the bloodstream, and helps to clear out mental blockages, freeing us up to be what we want to be. |
| Helpful foods | Blue and violet fruits, and vegetables such as purple broccoli. |

**VIOLET Ray**

| | |
|---|---|
| Characteristics | Because violet controls the Crown Chakra, it can be very stimulating for the nervous system, and encourage artistic abilities. |
| Subjects prone to | Mental and nervous disorders, neuralgia, sciatica. Any diseases of the hair and scalp. |
| As a treatment | Too much violet can cause out-of-body experiences, or not being fully in the body, so moderation in all things. Because violet cleanses venous blood, it is also very good for kidney and bladder problems. |
| Helpful foods | Aubergine, purple broccoli, purple grapes, blackberries. |

# Strengthening the Meridians Using Colour

Meridians are pathways in the body that relate to different organs. Acupuncturists will use these pathways to help with healing. With their sensitive touch, they will often sense areas within the body where energy is weak. As they insert an acupuncture needle into this area, it helps the body's energy to be renewed. This process has been described as like having two broken ends of energy along the meridian, and as the very fine acupuncture needle is inserted along this line, it joins the two ends together.

Often the person receiving this treatment will feel a surge of energy moving along this area. Sometimes the acupuncturist will use a substance called Moxa, which when set alight and smouldering, is held over the weakened area. The heat generated will often have the same effect as the needle.

When working with the Emotional Stress Release, there will be times when you are clearing the emotional blocks, and using the Finger Modes. From time to time it will centre on 'Electrical Circuits' finger mode, which is the thumb and little finger. This finger mode relates to the acupuncture meridians, or the electrical pathway to the organs of the body. This may indicate that there could be a certain part of the body that is in a weakened state, because of the emotions. Sometimes this is difficult to clear using the arm movements.

To strengthen, firstly you will need to dowse over the 'Meridian Charts' (see over) to find which meridian is at fault. When you have found the meridian that needs attention, note in which direction the tiny arrow is pointing on the meridian. Then dowse over the coloured felt tip pens to discover which colour you will need to use to balance this meridian.

So, for example, suppose you are clearing the feeling of ANGER from the age of 26, and although it has cleared from the electrical circuits, you do not get a strong response when you asked *"has it cleared?"* You can ask :

   *"Can I use colour on the meridian to strengthen?"*

If the answer is a "Yes", proceed as follows. Let us say you dowsed that the 'Liver' meridian was at fault. Now dowse to see which colour you will need to use to strengthen. Let us say the colour is Yellow.

To start off, ask your partner to think of 'ANGER' at the age of 26, if they can think of a specific occasion when anger affected them. If they can, that would be helpful, but even if they can't remember, this procedure will still work. As your partner is thinking of this emotion, ask :

*"Is this thought weakening the system?"*

You will probably get a *"Yes"* answer. Now still thinking of 'ANGER' at 26, put the yellow felt pen into their hand, and ask again :

*"Is this thought weakening the system?"*

You will find that this will now come up as a *"No"*, which often amazes people. When you take the felt pen out of their hand, and get them to think of ANGER again as you dowse and ask, the meridian will weaken again.

What you will do now is even more amazing. Go to the Liver on the meridian charts (see over). Take your yellow pen, *and with the lid firmly on your pen, so that you are not actually marking the paper,* and starting at the small arrow where the meridian begins at the big toe, run the pen along the path of the meridian three times. Repeat this on the other leg in the same direction, as the meridian is repeated on the other side of the body too.

Now ask your partner to think of ANGER again at 26, and ask :

*"Is the thought weakening the system?"*

This will now respond as *"No"*, even though your partner is not holding the yellow pen. It will have strengthened the body, by using the chart only.

# Meridian Charts

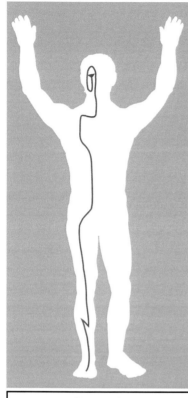

Stomach

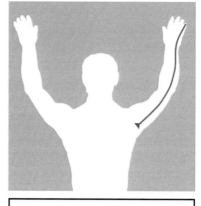

Heart

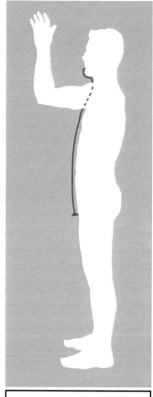

Central

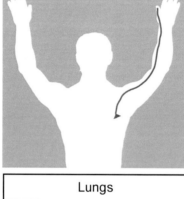

Lungs

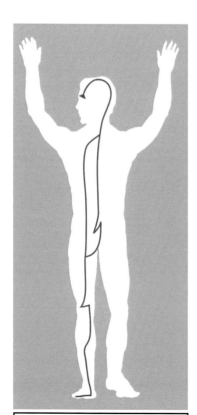

Bladder

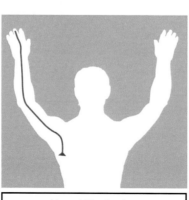

Heart Protector

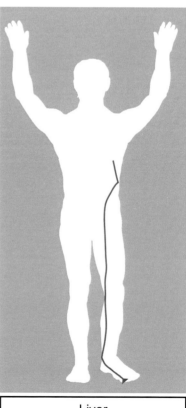

Liver

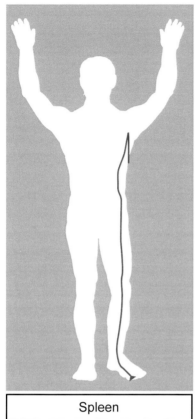

Spleen

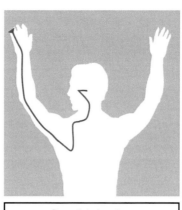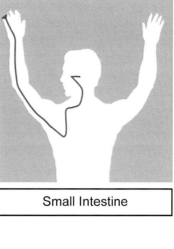

Small Intestine

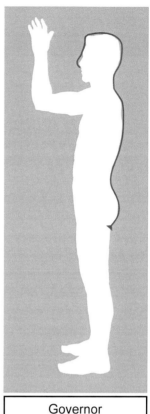

Governor

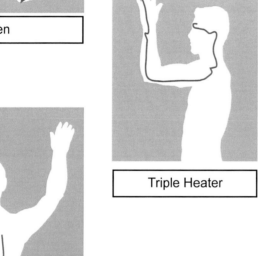

Triple Heater

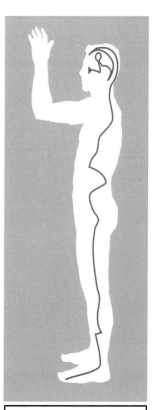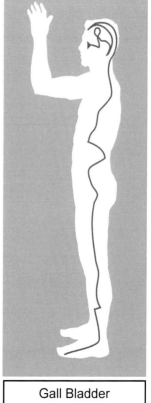

Gall Bladder

Kidney

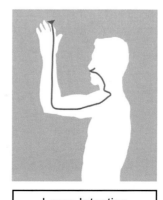

Large Intestine

# The Meridians

**STOMACH**

Health issues — The stomach carries out the first part of the process of receiving food and drink into our body, and transforming this into energy. It is responsible for the entire food pathway from the saliva in our mouth, down through the oesophagus and into the stomach and duodenum. If this does not function properly, symptoms such as indigestion, belching, obesity, ulcers and bowel problems will occur, and a general lack of vitality will be experienced.

Helpful foods — Vitamin B as in wheatgerm, wholegrains, liver, brewers yeast. It is also very important that food is chewed well.

Foods to avoid — Acidic foods, such as fizzy drinks, coffee, onions, tomatoes.

**HEART**

Health issues — One of the heart's main functions is to govern the blood and the entire functioning of the vascular system. It is not uncommon for patients who have issues of heart dysfunction such as palpitations or arrhythmia, to be told by their doctors that their heart is 100% sound. The heart also has a particular connection with the tongue and the ability to speak. Various speech defects, such as stuttering or even just tripping over one's words, can often be treated on the heart meridian.

Helpful foods — Calcium, Vitamins E and B, dairy foods, green vegetables, peas, beans, nuts, buckwheat.

Foods to avoid — Fatty, over processed foods, and an over-consumption of alcohol.

**SPLEEN**

Health issues — Closely linked with the stomach, and assists in the transformation of food and drink into blood. It also distributes energy around the body, so poor circulation and heavy-feeling limbs are often the result of a spleen dysfunction. Spleen controls the condition of the flesh and muscles. Many people find that under the stress of their busy lives, their muscle tone becomes increasingly tight. So aching limbs may be experienced.

Helpful foods — Vitamin A as in yellow and green peppers, as well as green leafy vegetables.

Foods to avoid — Refined sugar and other concentrated sweets, such as fruit juices.

**SMALL INTESTINE**

Health issues — Dysfunction of this meridian can cause many kinds of muscular-skeletal pain, such as frozen shoulder, stiff neck and tennis elbow. Digestive problems, hearing difficulties, tinnitus and urinary symptoms could also be affected. Physically, the small intestine is responsible for extracting what the body needs, and passing on to the large intestine what is not needed. It is responsible for receiving and making things thrive. In the mind and spirit, it performs the same function. The person may be stuck, or unable to commit themselves to a career or a relationship.

| | |
|---|---|
| Helpful foods | Vitamin B in yeast, wheat germ, yogurt, liver. |
| Foods to avoid | Bread, cakes, biscuits |

## BLADDER

| | |
|---|---|
| Health issues | The bladder meridian has the longest pathway in the body. Symptoms along its pathway are common, including headaches, back pains, sciatica and painful knees. Its main function is to control the distribution of fluids in the body, and it is closely linked with the kidneys. So cystitis and incontinence will be experienced when it malfunctions. |
| Helpful foods | Peas, beans, wheat germ, whole grains, raw fruit, cabbage, egg yolk, yeast. Also calcium in the form of dairy products, green leafy vegetables, beans, and nuts. |
| Foods to Avoid | Foods containing oxalic acid (cranberries, coffee, chocolate, purple fruits, particularly at meals where calcium is being consumed). |

## HEART PROTECTOR, OR CIRCULATION-SEX

| | |
|---|---|
| Health issues | The function is similar to the heart. The pericardium, the fibrous sheath that surrounds the heart, is governed by the heart protector. It is said that it guides the person in their joys and pleasures. It controls the person's ability to open and close their heart according to the needs of the situation. It protects the heart physically and it also protects emotionally, and in health, gives the person the necessary resilience to suffer the inevitable 'slings and arrows' of life. Some people with damaged heart protectors have closed their hearts to such an extent as to make it virtually impossible for them to enjoy an intimate relationship. |
| Helpful foods | Vitamin E and Zinc, green leafy vegetables, wheat germ, wholegrain cereals, eggs. |
| Foods to avoid | Acidic foods, such as onions, tomatoes and citrus fruits. |

## KIDNEYS

| | |
|---|---|
| Health issues | Problems with this organ may cause the person to have poor constitutional health. They may suffer problems such as retarded growth, premature ageing, or a weakness of sexual activity. The kidneys play a major role in the control of fluids in the body. There may be dark, scanty urine, constipation, dry mouth at night, as well as night sweats. There could also be an abundance of clear urine, oedema and loose stools. The condition of the bones and bone marrow is largely dependent on the kidneys. Brittle and soft bones as well as poor teeth are commonly seen when this organ is in poor condition. |
| Helpful foods | The need to drink large quantities of water on a regular basis cannot be emphasised enough. 2 litres per day is recommended. Kidney meat, vitamin A and E as in parsley, green pepper. All |

|                  | green leafy vegetables, wheat germ and green peas. |
|------------------|----------------------------------------------------|
| Foods to avoid   | Coffee and other strong beverages.                 |

## GALL BLADDER

| Health issues | This organ functions like the liver. Its dysfunction commonly results in problems with digestion, menstruation and the eyes. Painful shoulders, headaches, arthritis, particularly in the hips and knees are frequently the result of distress along the Gall Bladder meridian. Many people who have gall bladder problems, become clumsy and accident-prone, especially women around the time of their period. |
|---------------|---|
| Helpful foods | Vitamin A, green leafy vegetables, parsley (very similar to liver). |
| Foods to avoid | Fried foods, sugars and sweets, carbonated drinks and caffeine. |

## TRIPLE HEATER

| Health issues | No physical organ is associated with this meridian. It acts for the opening up of passages and irrigation, and as a thermostat in the body, regulating body temperature. |
|---------------|---|
| Helpful foods | Seaweed (Kelp) or lightly cooked fish. |
| Foods to avoid | Meat, especially if it has been processed, and shellfish. |

## LUNGS

| Health issues | The lungs govern the breath, and they are commonly treated when a person suffers from symptoms such as asthma, bronchitis or other lung problems. Lungs also govern the condition of the skin. |
|---------------|---|
| Helpful foods | Vitamin C in the form of green peppers and kiwi fruit. Citrus fruit too, just as long as it is fully ripe. |
| Foods to avoid | Mucous forming foods, such as dairy produce, sweets and chocolates |

## LIVER

| Health issues | Liver is responsible for the functioning of the eyes. Blurred vision, floaters in front of the eyes, dry, sore, tired or red eyes are all associated with the liver. When the Liver Meridian starts to malfunction, digestive disorders are very common. These include indigestion, nausea, flatulence and other kinds of digestive troubles. Digestive disorders are often brought on by eating in a tense manner, or by eating foods that the liver finds hard to deal with, such as rich, fatty foods. The liver is important in association with many types of menstrual problems, such as painful periods, fluid retention and premenstrual syndrome. Anger is the emotion associated with the liver. Arthritis and headaches may also be experienced, especially if there is an excessive consumption of alcohol, chocolate, drugs, cheese, and citrus fruits, to name a few. |
|---------------|---|

| | |
|---|---|
| Helpful foods | Vitamin A, green leafy vegetables, parsley. |
| Foods to avoid | Fried foods, sugars and sweets, alcohol, carbonated drinks. |

## LARGE INTESTINE

| | |
|---|---|
| Health issues | The large intestine is responsible for the elimination of waste from the body.  It is most important that the large intestine is functioning correctly, otherwise the body, mind and emotions will all be clogged, and toxic matter builds up. Constipation, diarrhoea, lower abdominal pain and flatulence are very common when this organ becomes out of balance. The large intestine also discharges waste material through the skin. Spots, blocked pores and greasy skin can all result when it malfunctions. Problems with the throat and nose, such as catarrh, sinus trouble and impaired sense of smell may also arise. |
| Helpful foods | Increased water intake, yogurt, honey, green vegetables and fruits. |
| Foods to avoid | Wheat products, over-consumption of red meats. |

## CENTRAL

| | |
|---|---|
| Health issues | This Meridian is associated with the arms and shoulder muscles. People that do a lot of thinking, or working at a desk, or do a lot of driving will often suffer from brain fatigue, and arms and shoulder stiffness. Sometimes this will show up in children who are slow learners. Trying to be as stress free as possible, will help this Meridian. Making sure that  these people get enough sleep, and do not skip breakfast, or do not eat in a hurried way, is very important.  Some simple stretching exercises would help the stiffness of muscles. |
| Helpful foods | Protein foods with plenty of vegetables and fruits. A good quality vitamin B Complex would help the nervous system. |
| Foods to avoid | Too many grains in the form of wheat. Limit fats and sugars, as acid foods create stress. |

## GOVERNOR

| | |
|---|---|
| Health issues | This Meridian is very similar to the Central Meridian, as it affects the neck and shoulder muscles, and problems could be caused by stress or bad seating. If this Meridian comes up as needing attention very often, it would be wise to visit a chiropractor as there may be a need for spinal adjustments. Some simple stretching exercises would be helpful for the stiffness. Neck problems can be associated with a pillow that is too high. |
| Helpful foods | Protein foods such as meats, fish, eggs could be of help. |
| Foods to avoid | Acid foods in the form of fats and sugars. Limit wheat products, and processed foods as these build up into acids, which are not good for the muscles. |

# Cutting The Ties That Bind

Working with the Diagnostic Sheet may often indicate that 'relationships' need attention. Ask your partner if they know who this person could be. This might not always be who they first think it is. Dowse to find whether this person is a male or female. Ask whether it is a parent, child or another family relation. It could be a work colleague. When you have isolated who is involved, have a copy of the 'Cutting the Ties that Bind' diagram in front of you.

Notice that the pin figures on the diagram have a darkened area around each one, and on the outside of this is a large figure of eight that crosses in the middle of the two.

Put your partner's name under the first pin figure, and the name of the person you are cutting the ties with, under the second pin figure. Have your coloured felt tipped pens ready.

We all have habits and mannerisms that could upset others. Sometimes we work with people that have hang-ups or behaviour problems that could cause stress or offence in the work-place. We could have an overpowering brother or sister, mother or father, partner, or even a child that you sometimes think goes out of its way to upset you. By working with this diagram it will not in any way harm them or yourself, but on the contrary, could free them and yourself to create a more harmonious relationship.

So, with your copy of the 'Cutting the Ties That Bind' diagram in front of you, dowse to see what colours your partner needs, to change the situation. There could be up to three colours that may be needed. Then in the darkened area, draw a circle around the first pin figure in the colour(s) chosen. Now concentrate on the other pin figure. Get your partner to think about the person with whom that they need a better relationship. While they are doing this, dowse over the coloured pens again and find the ones that this other person needs. When these have been found, draw a circle in that colour(s) in the darkened area on the second pin figure, as you did before.

So, now you will then be looking at the diagram, with one, two or three colours surrounding each of the pin figures.

Now look at the outer figure of eight that surrounds the two pin figures, with the centre of the eight crossing in the centre. Get your partner to mark over this figure of eight with a pen or pencil, as many times as they wish, following the lines of the figure of eight. They may want to take it home with them, and continue to do this, until they feel that they have done 'enough.'

Your partner then needs to cut through the centre of the eight, where it crosses over, so they now have two pieces. Each of these pieces need to be burnt, or destroyed in some way. It is important that they do not hold onto either of these pieces of paper, otherwise it will signify that they still want to hang onto past difficulties.

I have had quite a lot of positive feedback with this exercise. I was working with Miss A who has an inherited disability that causes problems from time to time. In the workplace, she gets on very well with many members of staff, but one lady in particular seemed to resent the fact that Miss A had to have time off occasionally, caused by her disability. This caused a lot of stress for Miss A, as it was something that she had no control over. After doing this exercise, the whole picture changed. The lady in particular suddenly became more helpful, began smiling more, which certainly released the tension, and my client became more confident.

**Cutting The Ties That Bind diagram**

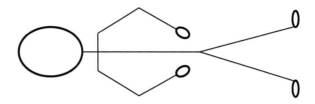

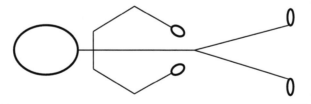

# Sounds

Sounds can be gentle and soothing, or brisk and exciting. Sound can lull us to sleep, or wake us up with fear and anxiety. Everyday sounds, like telephones, traffic noise, machinery, or pop music can often have a detrimental effect on the mind and body. The softer sounds within nature, such as bird song, the wind rustling the leaves on the trees, the hum of bees and insects, and the sounds of the sea as it ebbs and flows will be more positive. We are enveloped by sounds, and all of them have some effect on our mind or body.

Some sounds may be connected to past events, and emotions. Being a war child, I find even now, hearing an aircraft flying overhead in a slow laborious way, will still turn my stomach over. Hearing a police car in the road outside, reminds me of the anxious wait I had when one of our sons had not returned from his motor bike journey, only to get that fearful knock on the door, telling us that he was in hospital.

But of course, I do have other experiences of sound. I love to hear the first bumble bee of spring, the patter of rain on the window knowing that I am in the warm and dry. Summers on the beach, and the sounds of excited children. Other people have their own favourite sound.

Gentle music can softly lift a mood, or release tiredness. It can often surprise us by bringing tears to our eyes, whilst a bouncy tune can make us dance.

Certain notes actually link in with various parts of the body, and can have a dramatic healing effect. There are many people practising toning who find that it can have a huge calming affect on the nervous system, which in turn, helps to heal organs of the body.

Whilst I was recovering from an operation, a friend said she would send me some distance healing. She asked me to be still at a certain time, and told me that she would be 'toning'. I relaxed on the couch at the time designated, as asked. I was amazed, because I could definitely feel something going through my body, almost as if I was being touched by unseen hands.

There is much power in sound. An opera singer can break a glass just by singing a certain note. A marching army must break step over a bridge, as the sound and rhythm of their stride may upset the structure of the bridge, and it could collapse.

I know a school teacher with a class of very unruly boys. She has Mozart playing in the background and finds that the students respond greatly to this music. They calm down and are more attentive, which in turn produces better work.

Apparently, cows produce more milk if classical music is played in the milking parlour. Music has been known to make plants grow faster. So, it would seem that sound can affect other realms.

Jonathan Goldman, a leader in sound therapy, writes about toning in a dark place, at the base of a temple. As he was well into the toning, he became aware that this dark place became illuminated. His research led him to reach the following conclusion : through the use of vocally created harmonics it is possible to stimulate the pineal gland to produce light, which radiates out through the subtle body.

Coming from a Yoga background, I have used and experienced chanting, and the use of mantras, for calming the mind, and helping to focus. There will be many people who will have chanted the AUM Mantra, and experienced the tremendously uplifting effects, particularly if it is performed with a group of others. The AUM Mantra is called the universal sound. It brings us to the state of supreme awareness. Some may know the sound as OM, but by pronouncing AUM as three sounds, representing, the body, mind and spirit, it takes us deeper into a meditative state, linking us with our Higher Consciousness.

Dowse over the differing sounds, and find out which one is beneficial for your body. You can also dowse to find out how many times you need to perform this sound, and for how many days, weeks, or months.

When I am driving somewhere, I often make my mantra sounds. Nobody can hear me, so I do not get any funny looks.

| Mantra | Pronunciation | Benefits for ... |
|--------|---------------|------------------|
| 1. ee | as in **bee** | Upper skull |
| 2. ea | as in **feather** | Throat |
| 3. ah | as in **are** | Upper chest & lungs |
| 4. aw | as in **law** | Middle chest & lungs |
| 5. oh | as in **mow** | Heart, liver & stomach |
| 6. ue | as in **Debussy** | Kidney |
| 7. ir | as in **dirt** | Diaphragm, liver, Stomach |
| 8. ooee | as in **cooee** | Rectum |
| 9. ah ee | as in **car** and **feed** | Heart |
| 10. hr | as in **hurry** | Chest & lower throat |
| 11. fram | as in **fram** | Asthma, bronchitis |
| 12. hrm | as in **her-room** | Throat, nose, lung |
| 13. hrine | as in **her-rine** | Kidney |
| 14. hrown | as in **her-own** | Rectum |
| 15. hroom | as in **her-room** | Liver |
| 16. A U M | as in **ah oo mmmmm** | Relaxation for the Mind Body and Soul |

# Energy Transference

We are constantly being threatened, that our valued remedies from the healthfood shop, and our homeopathic pills, will no longer be available to us. This is a very sad situation, and very worrying. To make sure that you still have your own supply of your favourite remedies, you can use the Energy Transference and Neutralise Charts.

You need to purchase Sugar Pills, which can be obtained from a homeopathic supplier.

To use Energy Transference, place your chosen remedy, such as a tissue salt or homeopathic remedy on the Input ring shown below, and place the bottle containing sugar pills onto the Output ring.

Make a large circle with the pendulum, over the whole of the diagram with your remedies on it, until the pendulum changes direction. You will now have the remedy chosen, absorbed into the sugar pills. Take the dosage as previously prescribed.

If you wish, you can also transfer your remedy into a glass of water. In this case put your remedy onto the Input ring and place the glass of water onto the Output ring instead. If you choose this method of taking your remedy, only the right amount of the remedy will transfer to the glass of water.

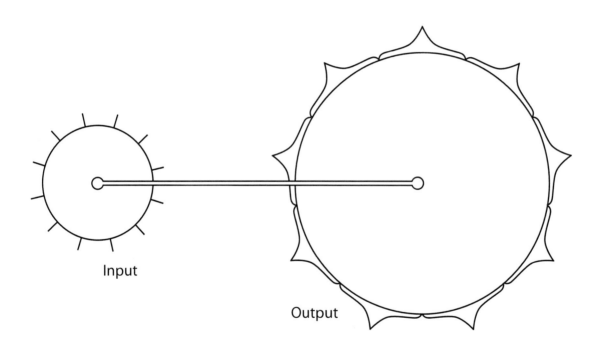

Input

Output

# Neutralise

To use the Neutralise facility, place the sugar pills to be neutralised in a sterile bottle on the centre of the Neutralise Chart. Set your pendulum swinging in a circular movement over the chart with your bottle of pills until the pendulium changes direction. This will remove any negative energy which may have occurred when handling them.

If you have any out-of-date tissue salts or homeopathic pills, these can be placed on the Neutralise diagram too, and will also remove anything that should not be there.

You can now use these pills for new remedies.

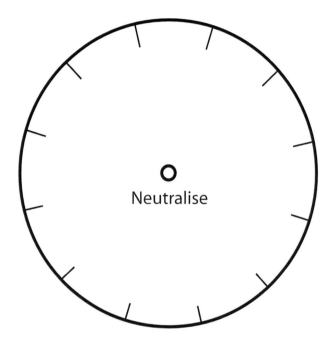

# Not The End

In the beginning I showed you how we can influence the pendulum by concentrating on the outer edges of the diagram, and how it altered the swing of the pendulum (see section: How The Mind Can Influence The Pendulum). Here is another exercise showing how the mind can influence things.

I want you to stand facing several metres of ground or floor in front of you. Walk in a straight line over this area, with your pendulum swinging in a neutral position (backwards and forwards). Do this for the length that you walk. Now go back to the beginning again. Walk halfway along the space you walked before, and this time mentally draw a straight line across the path that you have walked. I think of my index finger as being a marker and I use it as I would a chalk, raised high above the ground.

Stand at the beginning again and dowse as before along that path. You will notice that it changes direction over the area you have mentally marked and will continue into neutral once you have passed over the area. Please remember to rub out the line after you have done the exercise as this could be tripped over.

This exercise never ceases to surprise people, but shows very clearly that if we have negative thoughts about ourselves or our surroundings, how much we can be the cause of negativity in our life, even in a destructive way. In the same way, we can think and act in a positive way and overcome huge obstacles, which amaze us when we look back. *"How on earth did I do that"* you may say afterwards. There are many people in history who have performed the impossible, just because they believed that they could.

Many years ago I was introduced to an Indian therapy called Sanjivini, whereby shapes and symbols are projected into water or sugar pills for healing. I found that they worked in a wonderful way. On one occasion, a friend rang me from America and asked me what she could do for cystitis, and could I send her some absent healing. I said that I would, and dowsed over my Sanjivini charts. My pendulum swung very strongly over the diagram for the bladder and cystitis, but it also picked up on a fungal infection too, so I thought that maybe the problem causing the cystitis was a fungal outbreak. Several days later, my friend telephoned me and thanked me for the healing. Her cystitis had gone, but she was really surprised that a ringworm that she had on her leg for years had just broken up. Unbeknown to me, that was what the fungal infection was about, and the symbol had cleared that too.

I began to use the Sanjivini diagrams on my courses, but there were so many of them that photocopying them for each person on the course was a mammoth task. I considered dropping this form of healing from my courses, which was a shame as the diagrams worked very well, and can still be downloaded from the internet. I was pondering what to do next, when I remembered a fascinating book I read a few years back. The book is called *'The Hidden Messages in Water'* written by a Japanese writer called Masaru Emoto.

I had seen a previous book of his called *'The Messages of Water'* which consisted of a series of photographs that this man had taken showing ice crystals that had been made up from water that had been collected from many places. If the water was polluted, the ice crystals were shown as being badly deformed, and if it was from a healthy source, the ice crystals had a perfectly beautiful shape.

In his later book, Masaru Emoto had developed this further by putting water in a bottle and labelling it with positive or negative words. Amazingly, this changed the crystals too.

I decided to experiment with this. Using water that I had taken from a small bottle of spring water, I poured this into two other smaller bottles and labelled them, one with 'hate' on it and the other with 'love' on it. I left them overnight, and tasted them the following morning. 'Love' was sweet to the taste, but 'hate' tasted bitter, and I could not finish drinking it. As the two bottles had originally been from the same source, and just by attaching different words to the two bottles, there was now a significant change in the taste between them.

In 'The Hidden Messages In Water' Masaru Emoto describes an experiment that was performed by a family. Cooked rice was placed into two glass jars, and every day for a month, the family said *"Thank you"* to one jar, and *"You fool"* to the other jar. Even the children of the family did this too when they returned from school each day.

After one month, the rice that was told *"Thank you"* had started to ferment, with a mellow smell. The other jar with *"You fool"* said to it had rotted and turned black.

A later experiment was performed, using three jars of cooked rice. Two were made up as before, but the other jar was just ignored. The rice that had been ignored actually rotted before the rice that had been exposed to *"You fool"*, so the message here is that being ridiculed is actually not as damaging as being ignored. In his book, Masaru Emoto says :

> *"To give your positive, or negative, attention to something is a way of giving energy. The most damaging form of behaviour is withholding your attention."*

He also says :
> *"Gaze has a special energy of its own. A gaze of good intention will give courage, and an evil gaze will take it away."*

He also showed words to water, by wrapping a piece of paper with *"Love and Gratitude"* written on it. When frozen, the ice crystal was as perfect as could be, and produced a beautiful photograph. This suggests that Love and Gratitude are fundamental to the phenomenon of life in all nature. So perhaps we can use this for a simple, but effective form of healing.

The way we act and speak to others has influence. In another quote from this incredible book Masaru Emoto says :
> *"The vibrations created by Irritation are equivalent to those of Mercury, by Anger to those of Lead, and to those of Sadness and Sorrow to those of Aluminium. In the same way, Uncertainty is related to Cadmium, Despair to Steel and Stress to Zinc."*

He points out that Aluminium may be a contributing factor in Alzeimer's Disease, and if this is true, then it is likely that it is because Aluminium has the same vibrational frequency as Sadness, and so the sadness and sorrow of old age calls out to Aluminium, leading to the onset of Alzeimers.

So the possibilities of labelling a bottle of water with something like "Love and Gratitude" or "I am Sorry" or "Wisdom" or by standing the water on a picture of a spiritual place, or even exposing it to classical music can also be a tremendous healing remedy. Why am I telling you all of this and where is it leading? I am trying to show you that there is still a huge amount for us to discover and to use. I have led you through these exercises, which, over a number of years have been presented to me, and I have used and developed them into the form that they are in now. I want you to continue this journey now as part of your own discovery and development, and maybe developing the things that I have presented to you. In the words of Masaru Emoto :

> *"I think we underestimate the innate abilities that we each have; we have enormous power."*

My own personal words to you now are :

> *"The time is now."*

# Bag of Jewels

## Sayings by Famous People

*The worst thing you can possibly do is worry about what you could have done.*
- Lichenberg

*80% of success is just showing up.*
- Woody Allen

*Whenever we communicate with each other correctly, there is an exchange of energy.*
- Reshad Field

*Fear..the best way out is through.*
- Helen Keller

*Live as you will have wished to have lived when you are dying.*
- Gellert

*It's never too late to have a happy childhood.*
- Tom Robbins

*If you are going through hell, keep going.*
- Sir Winston Churchill

*What we see depends mainly on what we look for.*
- John Lubbock

*Life is a mirror and will reflect back to the thinker what he thinks into it.*
- Ernest Holmes

*Our minds can shape the way a thing will be, because we act according to our expectations.*
- Federico Fellini

*Change your thoughts and you change your world.*
- Norman Vincent Peale

*When patterns are broken, new worlds emerge.*
- Tuli Kupferberg

*These are my opinions and if you don't like them, I have others.*
   - Groucho Marx


*He who sees a need and waits to be asked for help is as unkind as if he had refused it.*
   - Dante Alighieri


*Happiness is experienced when your life gives you what you are willing to accept.*
   - Ken Keyes Jr.


*Two thirds of help is to give courage.*
   - Irish proverb


*Our business in life is not to get ahead of other people, but to get ahead of ourselves.*
   - Maltbie D Badcock


*We are rich, not according to what we have, but according to what we are.*
   - Anon


*You will not be judged by medals, degrees and diplomas in life, but by your scars.*
   - Anon


*The journey of a thousand miles begins with just one step.*
   - Lao-Tse


*Most griefs are medicinal.*
   - Shakespeare


*Defeat is not bitter if you do not swallow it.*
   - Anon


*Everyone is good at something*
   - Alan Titchmarsh


*Don't criticise the dark - light a candle.*
   - Barbara Sidebottom


*Those who bring sunshine into the lives of others cannot keep it from themselves.*
   - Anon

*It is good to have an end to journey towards,*
*but it is the journey that matters in the end.*

Ernest Hemingway